24 Solar Terms Regimen And Dietotherapy

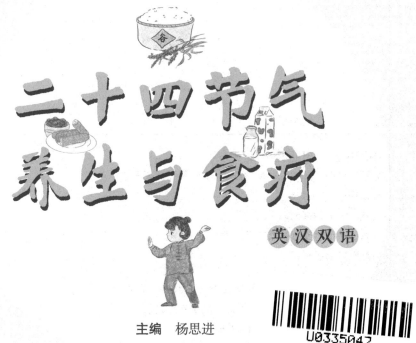

二十四节气 养生与食疗

英汉双语

主编　杨思进

Chief-compiler: Yang Sijir

副主编　徐厚平　汪建英

Deputy-compiler: Xu Houping, Wang Jianying

主译　李晓莉

Translated by Li Xiaoli

参译　温海煜　曹惜惜

Co-translated by Wen Haiyu & Cao Xixi

全国百佳图书出版单位
中国中医药出版社
·北京·

图书在版编目（CIP）数据

二十四节气养生与食疗 / 杨思进主编 . —北京：中国中医药出版社，
2022.1（2024.10重印）

ISBN 978 - 7 - 5132 - 7262 - 9

Ⅰ . ①二… Ⅱ . ①杨… Ⅲ . ①养生Ⅳ . ① R22

中国版本图书馆 CIP 数据核字（2021）第 069482 号

中国中医药出版社出版

北京经济技术开发区科创十三街 31 号院二区 8 号楼

邮政编码　100176

传真　010-64405721

北京盛通印刷股份有限公司印刷

各地新华书店经销

开本 710×1000　1/16　印张 11.25　字数 185 千字

2022 年 1 月第 1 版　2024 年10月第 2 次印刷

书号　ISBN 978 - 7 - 5132 - 7262 - 9

定价　48.00 元

网址　www.cptcm.com

服 务 热 线　010-64405510

购 书 热 线　010-89535836

维 权 打 假　010-64405753

微信服务号　zgzyycbs

微商城网址　https://kdt.im/LIdUGr

官 方 微 博　http://e.weibo.com/cptcm

天猫旗舰店网址　https://zgzyycbs.tmall.com

主编简介
Introduction of Chief-compiler
杨思进 Yang Sijin

杨思进，二级教授，博士研究生导师，国务院政府特殊津贴专家，全国中西医结合重点学科带头人，四川省中医药院士后备人才。国际中医药传承创新项目、国际中医临床研究基地建设项目、国家区域中医诊疗中心、国家中葡国际合作项目、国家商务部中医药服务出口基地、四川省博士后创新实践基地、四川省心脑血管研究中心负责人，岐伯生命健康文化研究院院长。

杨思进教授还担任世界中医药学会联合会急症专业委员会理事会副会长、中国中医药信息学会脑病分会会长、中国民族医药学会慢病管理分会副会长、中国民族医药学会脑病分会副会长、四川省中医药学会心脑血管病专委会主任委员、泸州市中西医结合学会会长等职务。

杨思进教授先后荣获全国郭春园式的好医生、中国百佳医院院长、最具影响力中国医院院长、四川省学术和技术带头人、四川省名中医、四川省有突出贡献专家、四川省卫生计生首席专家等殊荣。

杨思进教授从事医、教、研工作 30 余年，擅长运用中西医结合方法诊治心脑血管常见病、多发病及疑难重症。主持科研课题100 余项，发表学术论文 200 余篇，出版专著教材 40 余部，培养硕博士及博士后研究生 60 余名。

Prof. Yang is a Level-2 Professor (Professors in China fall into 4 levels) and doctoral supervisor with the following titles: The State Council Special Allowance Expert, Leader of National Key Disciplines of Integrative Chinese and Western Medicine, TCM Academician Reserve Talent of Sichuan Province, Director of International TCM Inheritance and Innovation Project, International TCM Clinical Research Base Project, International TCM Diagnosis and Treatment Center, Sino-Portuguese International Cooperation Project, Ministry of Commerce TCM Service Export Base, Postdoctoral Innovation and Practice Base of Sichuan Province, and Cardiovascular and Cerebrovascular Disease Research Center of Sichuan Province, as well as President of Qibo Institute of Life and Health Culture.

Prof. Yang holds the positions of Associate President of the Board of Directors of Emergency Committee of the World Federation of Chinese Medicine Societies, President of Encephalopathy Branch of China Information Association of Traditional Chinese Medicine, Associate President of Chronic Disease Management Branch of China Medical Association of Minorities, Associate President of Encephalopathy Branch of China Medical Association of Minorities, Chairman of Cardiovascular and Cerebrovascular Diseases Committee of Sichuan Association of Chinese Medicine, and President of Luzhou Society of Integrative Chinese and Western Medicine.

Prof. Yang has also been honored as one of the "Good Doctors like Guo Chunyuan", one of the Top 100 Hospital Directors in China, one of the Most Influential Hospital Directors in China, one of the Leading Academic and Technical Experts in Sichuan Province, one of the Leading TCM Practitioners in Sichuan Province, one of the Outstanding Experts in Sichuan Province, and one of the Leading Experts in Health Planning in Sichuan Province.

Prof. Yang has been engaged in medical, educational and research work for more than 30 years, specializing in the treatment of frequently-occurring or difficult-to-treat cardiovascular and cerebrovascular diseases by using integrative Chinese and Western medicine. He has presided over more than 100 scientific research projects, published more than 200 academic papers, more than 40 monographs and textbooks, and trained more than 60 postgraduates and postdoctoral students.

内容简介
Overview

本书结合立春、雨水、惊蛰、春分、清明、谷雨、立夏、小满、芒种、夏至、小暑、大暑、立秋、处暑、白露、秋分、寒露、霜降、立冬、小雪、大雪、冬至、小寒、大寒二十四节气，紧密联系生活实际，从饮食、睡眠、活动、穴位按摩等方面介绍了日常养生小知识。书中介绍的养生方法简单易行，养生食疗也便于取材。

本书图文并茂，语言通俗易懂，适合普通大众阅读。

This book introduces the 24 solar terms of the four seasons, i.e. Beginning of Spring (Lichun, 立春), Rain Water (Yushui, 雨水), Insects Awakening (Jingzhe, 惊蛰), Spring Equinox (Chunfen, 春分), Fresh Green (Qingming, 清明), Grain Rain (Guyu, 谷雨), Beginning of Summer (Lixia, 立夏), Lesser Fullness (Xiaoman, 小满), Grain in Ear (Mangzhong, 芒种), Summer Solstice (Xiazhi, 夏至), Lesser Heat (Xiaoshu, 小暑), Greater Heat (Dashu, 大暑), Beginning of Autumn (Liqiu, 立秋), End of Heat (Chushu, 处暑), White Dew (Bailu, 白露), Autumn Equinox (Qiufen, 秋分), Cold Dew (Hanlu, 寒露), First Frost (Shuangjiang, 霜降), Beginning of Winter (Lidong, 立冬). Light Snow (Xiaoxue, 小雪), Heavy Snow (Daxue, 大雪), Winter Solstice (Dongzhi, 冬至), Lesser Cold (Xiaohan, 小寒), and Greater Cold (Dahan, 大寒). Everyday activities are linked to how to cultivate health during these terms, including diet, sleep, exercises and acupressure. These methods are easy to learn and practice. Dietary recommendation is also convenient to try at home.

This illustrated book is highly recommended for the general public to read.

序
Preface

中医药学是中国古代科学的瑰宝，也是打开中华文明宝库的钥匙。千百年来，中医药学为中华民族的健康和繁衍作出了巨大贡献。中医药养生保健历经千年，已形成和积累了丰富的养生保健理论和经验。

Traditional Chinese medicine (TCM) is not only the treasure of ancient Chinese science but also the key to the treasury of Chinese civilization. Thousands of years have witnessed the tremendous contributions of TCM to the health and sustainment of the Chinese nation, as well as the development and accumulation of a wealth of theories and experiences in TCM health nurturing.

当今社会，随着人们的健康需求日益增长，中医养生也成了大家追逐的潮流。中医养生是指通过各种方法增强体质、预防疾病，从而达到延年益寿的目的，中医养生注重养生中机体的整体性和系统性。

With the increasing demand for health nowadays, TCM health nurturing has become a focus of interest among the public. It involves different methods for the purpose of prolonging life by strengthening physique and preventing diseases, where emphasis is placed upon the holistic and systematic features of the body.

《二十四节气养生与食疗》结合日常生活，从饮食、睡眠、活动、穴位按摩等方面介绍了一年四季二十四节气养生知识，由多名长期在医院从事中医临床工作的专家指导行文，具有以下特点。

This book titled *24 Solar Terms Regimen And Dietotherapy* introduces the knowledge of health nurturing in the 24 solar terms of the year in terms of diet, sleep, activity and acupressure, which can be applied in daily life. With the guidance of a number of experts who have long been engaged in TCM clinical work in hospitals, the book is endowed with the following characteristics.

一，节气养生。该书介绍了二十四节气的由来和特点，并介绍了节气的养生小知识和食疗方，方法简单可行。

Firstly, health nurturing with solar terms. The book introduces the origin and characteristics of the 24 solar terms, as well as tips of health nurturing and diet therapy, which is simple and feasible.

二，穴位养生。该书介绍的穴位由针灸专家推荐，图文结合，穴位养生方法通俗易懂。

Secondly, health nurturing with acupoints. The relevant acupoints are recommended by experts of acupuncture and moxibustion. The introduction of illustrations to the book makes it much easier to understand.

三，自绘图片。该书所有图片为主编单位——西南医科大学附属中医医院根据内容绘制而成，图片形象生动，读来趣味十足。

Thirdly, feature of original illustrations. All the illustrations in the book are original contribution from the Hospital (T.C.M) Affiliated to Southwest Medical University (Main Compiling Unit) based on the content in a vivid and interesting way.

《二十四节气养生与食疗》突出“自我养生调病”，图文结合，通俗易懂，便于传播。

是为序！

This book *24 Solar Terms Regimen And Dietotherapy* highlights "self-health nurturing and disease prevention". It is an illustrated book with plain language and easy to understand and helpful for dissemination, to which this preface is made with delight!

田金洲教授
北京中医药大学东直门医院
Prof. Tian Jinzhou,
Dongzhimen Hospital, Beijing University of Chinese Medicine

前言
Foreword

《黄帝内经》最早提出了"治未病"的理念，强调未病先防、已病防变、瘥后防复等多个方面的内容，即预防重于治疗。

The concept of "treating disease before onset" is first proposed in *The Yellow Emperor's Inner Classic* (*Huangdi Neijing*), which emphasizes prevention before disease onset, development control of existing diseases, and relapse prevention after recovery, i.e., prevention is more important than treatment.

本书编写团队认为，养生之道主要有二：一是养生理念，二是养生方法。本书编写团队提倡在遵守自然规律的前提下，围绕"上医治未病，中医治欲病，下医治已病"的理念，强调因时因地因人的日常生活养生，从而达到修身养性、强身健体的目的。

According to the compiling team, there are mainly two aspects of nurturing health, including the health-nurturing ideas and their implementing methods. It is advocated that health nurturing, with the premise of complying with the laws of nature, should center on the concept that "the superior practitioners treat disease before onset, the common practitioners arrest the occurrence, and the mediocre practitioners treat the existing disease". Tailored methods should be adopted in daily life according to time, place, and individual to achieve the purpose of nurturing and strengthening the body.

本书主要结合立春、雨水、惊蛰、春分、清明、谷雨、立夏、小满、芒种、夏至、小暑、大暑、立秋、处暑、白露、秋分、寒露、霜降、立冬、小雪、大雪、冬至、小寒、大寒二十四节气，紧密联系生活实际，从饮食、睡眠、活动、穴位按摩等方面介绍了日常养生小知识。

This book introduces tips for health nurturing of daily life in 24 solar terms of Beginning of Spring (Lichun), Rain Water (Yushui), Insects Awakening (Jingzhe), Spring Equinox (Chunfen), Fresh Green (Qingming), Grain Rain (Guyu), Beginning of Summer (Lixia), Lesser Fullness (Xiaoman) and Grain in Ear (Mangzhong), Summer Solstice (Xiazhi), Lesser Heat (Xiaoshu), Greater Heat (Dashu), Beginning of Autumn (Liqiu), End of Heat (Chushu), White Dew (Bailu), Autumn Equinox (Qiufen), Cold Dew (Hanlu), First Frost (Shuangjiang), Beginning of Winter (Lidong), Light Snow (Xiaoxue), and Heavy Snow (Daxue), Winter Solstice (Dongzhi), Lesser Cold (Xiaohan), and Greater Cold (Dahan) from the aspects of diet, sleep, activities, and acupoint massage.

编写之际正是 2020 年新型冠状病毒肺炎疫情之时，编者根据防治工作经验编写了 "新型冠状病毒肺炎防疫小知识"，介绍了疫情期间 "宅" 家自我健康管理的方法、提高免疫力食疗方，以飨读者。本书自绘图片，内容通俗易懂，介绍的养生方法行之有效，愿读者通过阅读本书能增长养生保健知识，获取养生之道，延年益寿。

This book was compiled in 2020 during the outbreak of novel coronavirus pneumonia (NCP). Hence, the compilers have prepared "NCP Prevention Tips" based on their experiences in the prevention and treatment of the disease, introducing methods of self-health management at home during the pandemic, as well as dietary therapies to improve immunity. The original illustrations make the content easy to understand, and health-nurturing methods are also effective. We hope that this book can help the audience to increase knowledge of health nurturing, and prolong their lives.

本书在编写过程中，得到了本书编写团队所在单位同仁大力支持和帮助，特此表示感谢！限于水平与时间，书中如有不足，望广大读者批评指正。

We appreciate support and help from our colleagues in the process of compiling. Due to constraint of knowledge and limit of time, there might be some mistakes and flaws in this book, please don't hesitate to give us feedback to correct them.

杨思进

Yang Sijin

目 录
Contents

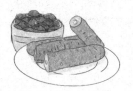
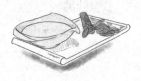

75/ 秋季 AUTUMN

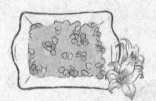

109/ 冬季 WINTER

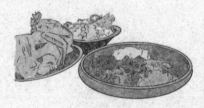

目录 CONTENTS

春季 SPRING

春三月，起于立春，止于立夏前，春季分为立春、雨水、惊蛰、春分、清明、谷雨六个节气。春季是冬季与夏季的过渡季节，冷暖空气势力相当，气温变化幅度大，空气干燥，多大风，北方多沙尘天气，南方多阴雨天气。春季人体皮肤毛孔舒张，对于外界的抵抗能力有所减弱。这时出门要注意防风，适当地"捂一捂"，年老体弱者尤应慎重。春季居处要注意室内卫生和开窗通风，同时，应避免冷风入室。

The three months of spring start with *Beginning of Spring* (Lichun) and end before *Beginning of Summer* (Lixia), with six solar terms of *Beginning of Spring*, *Rain Water* (Yushui), *Insects Awakening* (Jingzhe), *Spring Equinox* (Chunfen), *Fresh Green* (Qingming), and *Grain Rain* (Guyu) included. Spring connects winter and summer. It is featured by a matched rival between cold and warm air, big temperature change, dryness, frequent strong wind, and sandy weather in the north while rainy weather in the south. In such a season, the pores tend to open, which means decreased immunity against external pathogens. Consequently, wind should be kept away when going out, and appropriate "covering up" is recommended, especially for the elderly and the infirm. For the daily life, attention should be paid to indoor sanitation and ventilation, and at the same time, the cold wind should be prevented.

●宜：性味[1]微辛微温的食物，如葱、姜、蒜、韭菜和芥末等，以及富含蛋白质的食物，如鸡蛋、牛奶、鱼类和豆类等。

Recommended: Foods that are slightly pungent in property[1] and slightly warm in flavor, such as green onion, ginger, garlic, Chinese chives, mustard, etc.; and protein-rich foods, such as eggs, milk, fish, and beans, etc.

[1] 性味：指寒、热、温、凉四种；性味：指辛、甘、酸、苦、咸五种味。

[1] Property: cold, hot, warm and cool; Flavor: pungent, sweet, sour, bitter, and salty.

●不宜：牛肉、羊肉、鸽子肉及白酒、人参等大温大热的食物。春季饮食应掌握以下五大原则。

Not Recommended: Foods that are extremely warm or hot in property, such as beef, mutton, pigeon meat, Chinese liquor, ginseng and so on. Diet in spring should follow the five principles stated below.

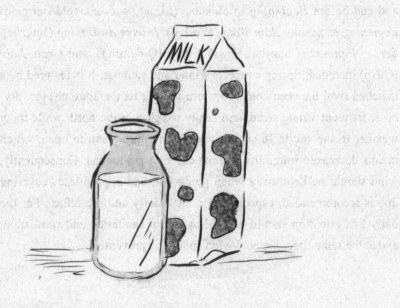

饮食

【多主少副】

多吃主食，少吃副食。春季风多雨少气候干燥，气温变化反复无常，人体免疫力和防御功能下降，易诱发一些春季常见的疾病。此时可以多吃些主食，其主要成分是碳水化合物，能够直接转化成热量，提供身体基本所需。同时，春季应注重调养肠胃，米饭相比较大鱼大肉，要容易消化，能更好地保护消化功能。

More carbohydrates, less heavy foods

Increase the intake of carbohydrates and decrease heavy foods. Spring is featured by frequent wind, little rainfall, dry air and unpredictable temperature change, and immunity of the body tends to decrease accordingly, which might induce some common diseases in spring. What is recommended is carbohydrates which can directly produce energy needed. At the same time, the spleen and stomach should be focused, and rice is more favored than fish and meat as rice is easier to digest and protective for digestive function.

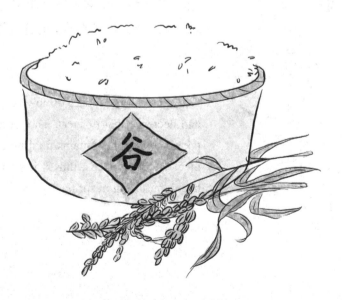

【多菜少果】

多吃蔬菜，少吃水果。春季以养肝为主，多吃富含维生素、纤维素和矿物质的蔬菜，如番茄、荠菜、黄瓜、萝卜等，有疏通血管和肠道的特殊功能。水果应适量，酸甜的水果中含有较多果酸，属生冷食物应少吃，如柑橘、柚子、山楂等。

More vegetables, less fruits

Increase the intake of vegetables and decrease that of fruits. In spring, emphasis should be placed upon nourishing the liver. Vegetables that are packed with vitamin, fiber, and minerals are recommended, such as tomato, shepherd's purse, cucumber, and radish, as they can dredge blood vessels and intestines. The amount of fruit intake should be appropriate, including fruits that are sour and sweet in flavor due to high acid content or cold in property, such as citrus fruits, pomelo, Chinese hawthorn fruit, etc.

【多奶少肉】

多喝牛奶或羊奶，少吃肉类。牛奶是全营养食物，春季多喝奶能满足人体需求，是各类人群春季养生的首选佳品。

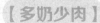

More milk, less meat

Increase the intake of cow or goat milk and decrease that of meat. The increased intake of milk that contains total nutrients can meet the body needs, thus it is preferred for health nurturing in spring.

【多水少油】

多补充水分，少吃油腻食物。冬春季节更替，常多风、干燥，加剧身体水分的流失，最简单的排毒方法就是多喝水，日饮水量 2000mL 左右，有助于清洗肠道。

More water, less oil

Increase the intake of water and decrease that of greasy food. The alternation of winter by spring often manifests as frequent wind and dryness which will accelerate water loss of the human body. Increased intake of water at about 2000 mL a day is recommended, which helps to detoxify the body and cleanse the intestines.

【多彩少单】

多吃五颜六色的食物，少吃颜色和口味单调的食物。五脏[1] 各有所爱，如心爱红、苦；肝爱绿、酸；肾爱黑、咸；肺爱白、辣；脾爱黄、甜。人们的饮食中，应当多照顾到各脏器的爱好。

More varieties in the colors of food

Increase the variety of diet color. In Traditional Chinese Medicine, five *zang*-organs[1] have their corresponding favorable colors and flavors. For example, heart favors redness and bitter; liver, green and sour; kidney, black and salty; lung, white and spicy; spleen, yellow and sweet. Attention should be paid to such relations of different *zang*-organs when it comes to diet.

[1] 五脏：①西医的"脏"是以人体局部解剖位置定位划分，五脏是指心脏、肝脏、肺脏、肾脏、脾脏，是单纯的五个脏器的统称；②中医的"脏"是以人体系统功能作用划分的，五脏是指心、肝、脾、肺、肾五脏系统的总和。

[1] Five *zang*-organs: ① Western medicine defines *zang* (viscera) according to their anatomical position in the body. The five viscera refer to the heart, liver, lung, kidney and spleen, which are the general name of the five simple organs; ② Traditional Chinese medicine defines *zang*-organs according to the function. "Five-*zang* organs" is a combination of systems of five *zang*-organs, including the heart, liver, spleen, lung, and kidney.

睡眠

【晚睡早起】

春季昼长夜短，天黑得晚、亮得早，应顺应自然规律，提倡晚睡早起。晚睡即把平时睡觉的时间稍微推后一点，每晚 23 时至次日 6 时是春季睡眠的最好时间。

Sleeping later and rising earlier

In spring when the days are long and the nights are short, it is recommended to adjust the routine accordingly and go to bed a bit later than usual and get up early. The time from 11 pm to 6 am of the next day is mostly suitable for sleep.

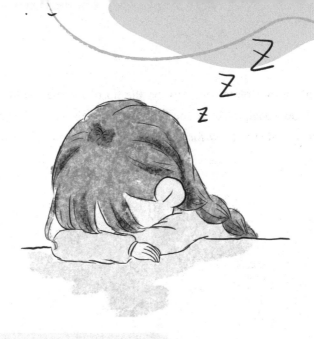

【缓解春困，可午休半小时】

春季容易"春困"，要缓解春困，午睡不可少，春季午睡时间应保持 15 ～ 30 分钟，时间过久则易越睡越困。

Taking a 30-minute nap after lunch in sleepy spring

People tend to feel sleepy in spring, for which a nap after lunch at about 15 to 30 minutes is necessary. Besides, prolonged nap does not contribute to refreshment.

【难以入睡，可揉搓涌泉穴】

涌泉穴位于足底部，蜷足时足前部凹陷处。难以入睡时，将一只脚的脚心放在另一只脚的大踇趾尖，来回做摩擦涌泉穴的动作，直到脚心发热，再换另一只脚。交替进行 10 ～ 15 分钟，有助于入睡。

Massaging Yongquan for difficulty in falling asleep

Yongquan (KI1) is located at the sole of the foot, and can be found in the anterior depression when flexed. When there is difficulty in falling asleep, place the sole of one foot on the tip of the big toe of the other foot, and rub Yongquan back and forth until it feels warm, then switch to the other foot alternatively for a total of 10 to 15 minutes, which helps to fall asleep.

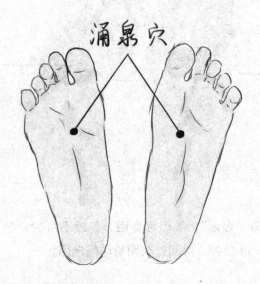

【早晨起床时多伸懒腰】

经过一夜睡眠后，人体松软懈怠，总觉懒散而无力。若四肢舒展，伸腰展腹，全身肌肉用力，并配以深吸深呼，可解乏、醒神。伸懒腰时要使身体尽量舒展，四肢要伸直，全身肌肉都要用力，时间控制为 3～5 分钟。

Stretching the body while getting up in the morning

Sleep over the night makes the body slack and lethargic. Combined with deep breathing, stretching the four limbs, waist and abdomen, and tensing the muscles of the body can relieve fatigue and make one feel re-freshed. When stretching, the body should be stretched as far as possible and the limbs should be straight for 3 to 5 minutes.

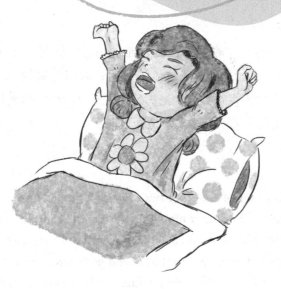

高血压、心脏病患者伸懒腰时，动作要慢且不要憋气；而腰椎疾病患者不适合伸懒腰。

For patients with hypertension and heart diseases, the stretching should be slow and holding breath should be avoided. What's more, this is not suitable for patients with lumbar diseases.

活动

春季气温仍较低，活动时要注意防风御寒，肢体不要过于裸露，以免造成关节的损伤。推荐以下几项养生活动。

The temperature is still low in spring. Be careful of the wind and cold during exercises, and avoid exposing the limbs directly in case joint injuries may happen. The following health-nurturing activities are recommended.

【放风筝】

放风筝是集休闲、娱乐和锻炼为一体的养生活动。风筝放飞时，人不停地跑动、牵线、控制，通过手、眼的配合和四肢的活动，可达到活动筋骨、强身健体的目的，时间控制为 30 ～ 60 分钟。中老年人放风筝时要注意保护颈部，不要后仰时间太长，可仰视和平视相交替，而有眩晕者不适合放风筝。

Flying kites

Kite-flying is a health-nurturing activity for entertainment and exercise. It involves constant running and controlling of the thread with coordination of hands and eyes and the movement of four limbs, through which muscles and bones are exercised and body strengthened. The duration is expected to be 30 to 60 minutes. For the middle-aged and the elderly, the neck should be protected when flying kites and longtime leaning-back is forbidden. Instead, they can look up at the sky and look at the front horizontally alternately. Those with vertigo are not suitable for flying kites.

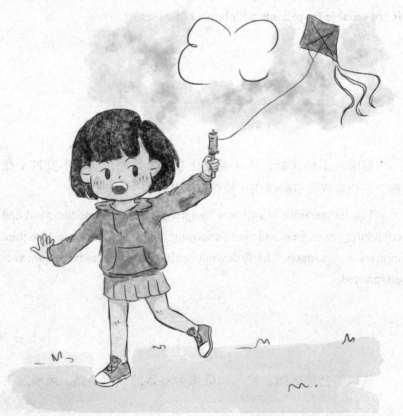

【打太极拳】

太极拳柔和、缓慢、刚柔并济，打太极拳不仅能改善肌肉及关节酸痛，还能通过呼吸与运动间的相互配合，达到强身健体的作用。打太极拳宜选择清晨的湖边、江边等空气清新的地方，时间控制为每次 20 ～ 30 分钟，但膝关节半月板损伤者，伤损未愈的情况下不建议打太极拳。

Practicing tai chi

Through gentle, slow and flowing movements, tai chi can not only improve pain in the muscle and joints, but strengthen the body with combination of movement and breathing. It is suggested to practice for 20 to 30 minutes each time by the lake in the morning when the air is fresh. However, it is not suitable for those with meniscus injury of knee joints.

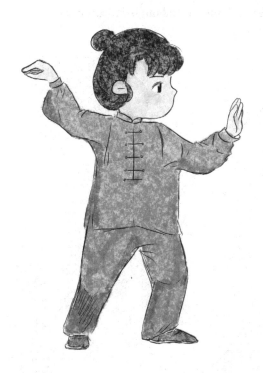

【垂钓】

春季温度渐升，水下的鱼群也变得活跃起来，适宜垂钓。垂钓能去除杂念、平心静气、舒缓神经，对于高血压、神经衰弱、消化不良者均有益处。垂钓应选择水面较小、水深在 1.5 米以下的坑塘或水面虽大但向阳的浅滩，如有水草或芦苇则更佳，时间控制为2～3 小时。腰椎疾病、颈椎病等患者不适宜长时间垂钓。

Fishing

With the rising temperature in spring, fish also becomes active, which is a good time for fishing. Fishing can help remove distracting thoughts and relax the mind, which is beneficiary to those with hypertension, nervous breakdown, and dyspepsia. The place for fishing can be either small ponds that are no more than 1.5 meters deep or large shallows that face the sun. Those with waterweeds or reeds are preferred. The time for fishing should be 2 to 3 hours. For those with lumbar diseases or cervical spondylosis, longtime fishing is inappropriate.

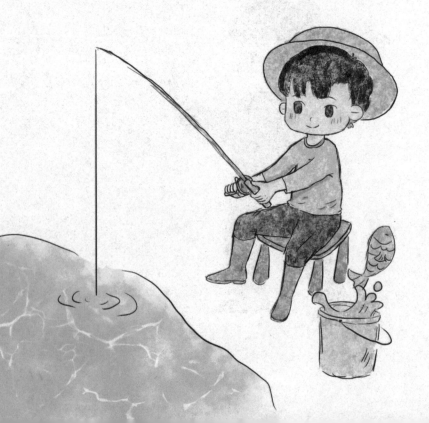

穴位养生

春季养生除了通过饮食、睡眠、活动的日常调养外，还可以通过穴位按摩达到养生之效。春季养生重在养肝，可通过以下穴位进行调护。

Health nurturing in spring involves not only daily adjustment of diet, sleep, and outdoor activities, but also acupoint massage. At this time, emphasis should be placed on nourishing the liver, for which the following acupoints can be selected.

大敦穴

【位置】位于大踇趾外侧的趾甲缝旁边。

【功效】清肝明目；使头脑清晰，神清气爽。

【方法】大敦穴可按摩，也可艾灸。可将艾绒[1]捏成麦粒状，放置于大敦穴上，点燃，待皮肤有温热感时将艾绒取下，再放置下一粒，每次5～7粒，每周1～2次。

Dadun (LR1)

Location: On the lateral side of the big toe, next to the corner of the nail.

Actions: Clearing the liver and improving vision; refreshing the mind.

Methods: Massage the acupoint or apply moxibustion. Knead the moxa floss [1] into cones like wheat seeds. Place the grain-shaped cone on the acupoint and ignite it. Replace the cone with another when the skin feels warm for a total of 5 to 7 cones each time, 1 to 2 times a week.

　　［1］艾绒：是由艾叶经过反复晒杵、捶打、粉碎，筛除杂质、粉尘，而得到的软细如棉的物品。

　　［1］Moxa floss: The soft and fine product is made of mugwort after repeatedly drying, pounding, crushing, and screening of impurities and dust.

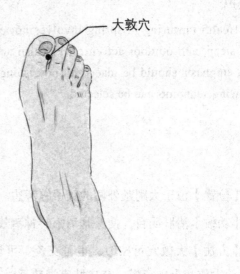

大敦穴

太冲穴

【位置】位于大踇趾缝往脚背上约 2cm 处。

【功效】能很好地调动肝经的元气，使肝脏功能正常，对调节血压也有较好功效。

【方法】每天晚上热水泡完脚后，用左手的大拇指点按右脚背上的太冲穴约 100 次，左侧亦然。

Taichong (LR 3)

Location: About 2 cm above the place where the skin of your big toe and the next toe joint.

Actions: Regulating qi of liver meridian to maintain normal liver function and regulate blood pressure.

Methods: Press the acupoint on the right foot with the thumb of the left hand about 100 times, and so does the left side, once every night after foot bath in warm water.

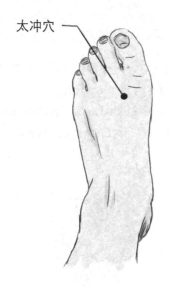

太冲穴

肝俞穴

【位置】位于背部脊椎旁边，第九胸椎棘突下，旁开 1.5 寸 [1]（取穴时，采用正坐的姿势，从低头时最高隆起处那块骨头算起，往下数第九个凸起，该凸起下方左右各两横指宽处，即为肝俞穴）。

【功效】对于各种肝胆性疾病具有一定调理作用。

【方法】坐位或俯卧位，双手拇指按压肝俞穴，按压时，一面缓缓吐气一面按压，直至局部有酸胀感为宜，每次按压约 10 分钟。

Ganshu (BL 18)

Location: 1.5 *cun* [1] lateral to the lower border of the spinous process of the 9th thoracic vertebra (When selecting the acupoint, the sitting position is adopted. Ganshu acupoints are located about 2 fingers width lateral to the lower border of the 9th bulge below the first bone at the highest bulge when the head is lowered.)

Actions: Regulating diseases of the liver and gallbladder.

Methods: Take sitting or prone position. Use both thumbs to apply pressure on the acupoints, and exhale slowly at the same time until there is distending and sore sensation. Each process should last for ten minutes.

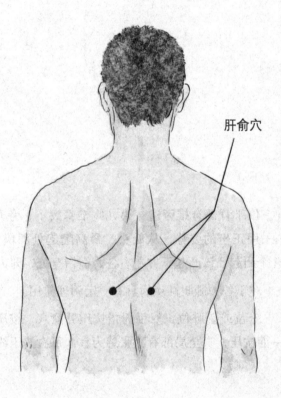

肝俞穴

立春 Beginning of Spring (Lichun)

立春为每年公历 2 月 5 日前后，太阳黄经为 315°。立春是二十四节气的第一个节气，我国习惯把它作为春季开始的节气。

Beginning of Spring (Lichun) usually falls around February 5th in Gregorian calendar of the year with the ecliptic longitude of 315°. It is the first of the 24 solar terms and lifts the curtain of spring.

【立春养肝为主】 Nourishing the liver in Spring

❶ 充分休息养肝

立春是细菌、病毒繁殖旺季，肝脏具有解毒、排毒的功能，负担最重，此时应充分休息，每天保证睡眠时间 6 小时以上，午休 30 分钟左右。

❶ Taking full rest

Beginning of Spring is the peak time of bacteria and virus proliferation, which imposes an extra load on the liver since it has the function of detoxification. Full rest, including no less than 6 hours' night sleep and about 30-minute nap at noon, should be maintained.

❷ 拒绝大怒护肝

肝喜欢心情舒畅，生气、发怒易诱发各种肝病，"怒伤肝"就是这个道理。所以，立春要尽量做到心平气和、乐观开朗，避免肝火太旺或肝气郁结，久而久之致肝病。

❷ Avoiding rage

The ease of mind favors the smooth flow of liver qi while anger tends to incur various liver diseases, which, in other words,

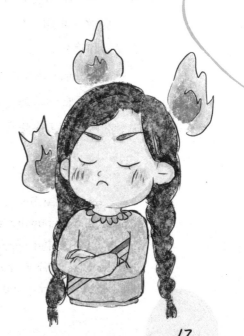

is "anger impairing the liver". Therefore, a good mood in the *Beginning of Spring* is important to avoid exuberant liver fire or stagnation of liver qi that will develop into liver diseases gradually.

❸ 慢跑运动卫肝

立春进行适当的户外慢跑运动，既能使气血舒畅，又能怡情养肝，每次建议控制在 1 小时以内。但肝病患者须注意不能过于劳累，每次最好控制在 30 分钟内。

❸ Jogging

Appropriate jogging outside in the *Beginning of Spring* contributes to not only smooth flow of qi and blood, but also a calm mind and thus nourishing the liver. It should be within one hour each time, while for those with liver diseases who should avoid exhaustion, the time can be decreased to 30 minutes.

【立春食疗方：胡萝卜炖牛肉】

材料：牛肉 250g，胡萝卜 120g，盐、胡椒粉、鸡精、酱油、葱、姜、蒜适量。

做法：牛肉焯水待用；凉水放入胡椒粉、酱油、葱、姜、蒜，开锅后放入牛肉，1 小时后倒入胡萝卜，炖约 30 分钟，出锅时放适量盐和鸡精。

功效：消除疲劳，增强体能。

适宜人群：一般人群均可食用。尤其适合体虚、筋骨酸软、贫血、久病、面黄头晕者。

Diet therapy: Stewed beef with carrots

Ingredients: Beef 250 g, carrots 120 g, appropriate amount of salt, pepper, chicken powder, soy sauce, green onion, ginger, and garlic.

Methods: Put pepper, soy sauce, green onion, ginger, and garlic into the water. When the water boils, add the blanched beef. One hour later add the carrots and stew for another 30 minutes. Add appropriate amount of salt and chicken powder when it is accomplished.

Actions: Relieving fatigue and strengthening the body.

Indicated population: General population, especially those with deficient constitution, weak bones and tendons, anemia, chronic diseases, as well as those with sallow complexion and dizziness.

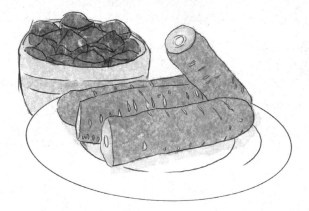

雨水 Rain Water (Yushui)

雨水为每年公历 2 月 19 日前后，太阳黄经为 330°。这时，春风遍吹、冰雪融化、空气湿润、雨水增多。人们常说："立春天渐暖，雨水送肥忙。"此时，人们开始备耕生产。

Rain Water (Yushui) occurs on around February 19th when the sun reaches the celestial longitude of 330°. In such a solar term, with the gentle spring wind comes the melting of snow and ice, increased rainfall, and moist air. There is an old saying that "While *Beginning of Spring* brings rising temperature, *Rain Water* facilitates the absorption of fertilizers". It is high time for preparation of plowing and production.

【雨水春捂更防病】Covering up to avoid diseases

❶ 不忙减衣

雨水到来，气温回升，但此时气温忽高忽低，天气忽冷忽热，容易患上感冒、支气管炎等疾病，也会使原有的疾病加重，故此时不宜过早地脱掉棉衣。

❶ Keeping wearing warm clothing

Temperature does rise in the *Rain Water*, but in an unstable manner. Such changeable weather makes it easy to contract diseases such as colds and bronchitis, and will also aggravate the original diseases. Therefore, it is recommended to keep wearing warm clothing.

❷ 上薄下厚

春季随着气温回升，机体活动度逐渐增强，一旦有冷空气入侵，易出现腰膝酸软、疼痛麻木等。雨水处于初春时节，下身的裤子、袜子、鞋子，一定要穿得厚点儿、暖和点儿，上身则可选择轻薄材质的衣服，如针织类外套。

❷ Less clothing in the upper body, more clothing in the lower body

Activities of the body gradually increase in spring as temperature rises. Once there is cold invasion, symptoms like soreness and weakness of the waist and knees as well as pain and numbness can occur. At the initial stage of spring, you should wear more in the lower part, such as trousers, socks and shoes that can keep warm, while for the upper body, light and thin clothing like knitted coat can be chosen.

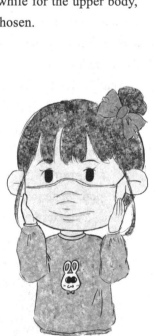

❸ 做好防护

雨水是春季常见病多发的节气，过敏性疾病尤为高发。特别是患有慢性支气管炎、哮喘、皮肤病者，出门要戴口罩，少去公共场合。

❸ Personal protection

Various diseases in spring, especially allergic diseases, tend to occur in *Rain Water*. For those with chronic bronchitis, asthma, and skin diseases, remember to wear a mask for outdoor activities, and avoid crowded public places.

【雨水食疗方：粉葛豆豉粥】

材料：粉葛 10g，淡豆豉 10g，葱白 3 茎，麦冬 10g，粳米 50g。

做法：将粉葛、淡豆豉、麦冬放入砂锅中，加水 500mL，置火上煮沸 5 ～ 10 分钟，滤去渣，于药汁中放入粳米，同煮为稀粥；将葱白洗净后切成段，于药粥将成时放入，搅拌即成；温服。

功效：健脾和胃，养阴生津。

适宜人群：肠胃功能不好所致的腹胀、解稀便、食欲不振、浑身无力、容易疲倦，以及口干、眼干者。

Diet therapy: Pueraria Root and Prepared Soybean Porridge

Ingredients: Pueraria root (Fenge) 10g, prepared soybean (Dan Douchi) 10g, green onion stalks 3 pieces, ophiopogon tuber (Maidong) 10g, japonica rice 50g.

Methods: Put pueraria root, prepared soybean and ophiopogon tuber into a casserole filled with 500 mL water. Heat the water and boil for another 5 to 10 minutes. Filter out the residue, and add japonica rice into the medicinal juice, and cook it as porridge. Wash the green onion stalks and cut them into sections, then put them into the porridge and stir. Take the porridge while it is warm.

Actions: Strengthening the spleen and harmonizing the stomach, nourishing yin and producing fluid.

Indicated population: Those with abdominal distension, loose stool, poor appetite, and lack of strength due to hypofunction of the stomach and intestines; and those with dry mouth and dry eyes.

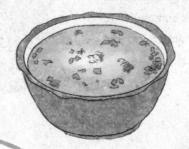

惊蛰 Insects Awakening (Jingzhe)

惊蛰为每年公历 3 月 6 日前后，太阳黄经为 345°。惊蛰时，天气转暖，春雷开始震响，蛰伏在泥土中的各种冬眠动物将苏醒过来开始活动。进入惊蛰后，人们便开始忙碌春耕了。

Around March 6th when the sun reaches the celestial longitude of 345°, the solar term of *Insects Awakening* (Jingzhe) begins. The solar term heralds warm weather and spring thunder. While animals are awakened from winter sleep, farmers are busy with spring plowing.

【惊蛰防六类疾病】Preventing six kinds of diseases

❶ 感冒和流感

惊蛰天气忽冷忽热，感冒和流感就成了常客，严重者甚至会引发气管炎、肺炎等疾病。

预防：老年人、儿童及体弱多病者尽量少去公共场所。易感冒者可每日早晚用淡盐水漱口；用姜末加红糖开水冲泡后，晚间睡前服用。

❶Colds and flu

Insects Awakening is featured by changeable weather, as a result of which colds and flu occur frequently, and in severe cases, bronchitis and pneumonia might be complicated.

Prevention: The elderly, children, and the infirm should avoid crowded public places. Those prone to colds should gargle with salt water every morning and evening; they can also drink ginger powder with brown sugar mixed with boiled water before sleep.

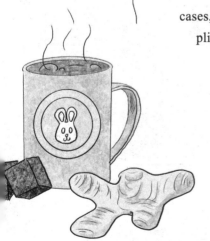

❷ 皮肤病

惊蛰天气转暖，皮肤的新陈代谢逐渐加快，皮脂和汗液的分泌逐渐旺盛。皮肤抵抗力降低，易过敏人群易出现发红、瘙痒、脱皮等症状。

预防：易过敏人群应减少与花粉、化妆品等的接触，可以吃一些预防过敏的食物，如红枣、山药、蜂蜜、胡萝卜等。

❷ Skin diseases

As the weather gets warmer in *Insects Awakening*, there is increase in skin metabolism and secretion of sebum and sweat. Therefore, those prone to allergies can develop redness, pruritus, peeling and other symptoms due to decreased skin immunity.

Prevention: Those prone to allergies should decrease contact with pollens and cosmetics, and eat jujubes, yam, honey, carrots, etc. that can prevent allergies.

❸ 肠胃疾病

惊蛰雨水渐多，易导致细菌和病毒滋长，胃肠疾病易乘虚而入。

预防：要注意饮食和个人卫生，不要吃生冷食物，食物尽量加热后食用。

❸ Digestive diseases

Increased rainfall in *Insects Awakening* might lead to proliferation of bacteria and virus, which makes it easier for digestive diseases to occur.

Prevention: Pay attention to diet and personal sanitation. Avoid cold and raw food and heat the food before eating.

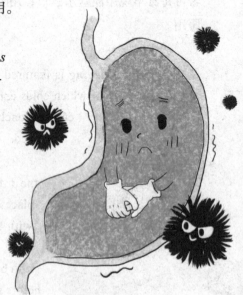

❹ 过敏性疾病

惊蛰开始，天气回暖，花粉、粉尘逐渐增多，极易诱发花粉症、支气管哮喘、过敏性鼻炎等过敏性疾病。

预防：避免与变应原接触，减少户外活动，随身携带抗过敏药物，有哮喘病史者发病须立即就医。

❹Allergic diseases

With the rising temperature in Insects Awakening comes increased pollens and dust in the air, which will induce allergic diseases, such as pollinosis, bronchial asthma, and allergic rhinitis, etc.

Prevention: Avoid contact with allergens and reduce outdoor activities. Carry antiallergic drugs with you. Those with history of asthma should go to hospital immediately upon onset.

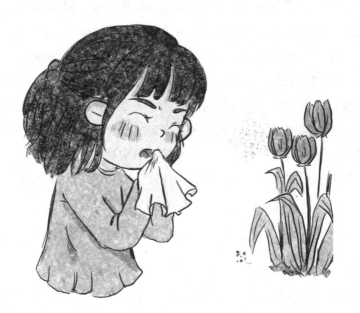

❺ 心脑血管疾病

惊蛰冷热不定，人体血管收缩情况也极不稳定，易导致血压不稳，从而引发高血压、脑血栓、中风等心脑血管疾病。

预防：老年人是心脑血管疾病高发群体，应提前做好预防，根据气温变化增减衣物，另外注意监测血压，保持心情舒畅。

❺Cardiovascular and cerebrovascular diseases

The blood pressure is unstable due to erratic vasoconstriction caused by changeable weather in *Insects Awakening*. Consequently, cardiovascular and cerebrovascular diseases such as hypertension, cerebral thrombosis and stroke, etc. might occur.

Prevention: The elderly are at high risk of cardiovascular and cerebrovascular diseases. Prevention of such diseases through dressing appropriately according to the temperature, monitoring blood pressure, and keeping an easy mind, should be emphasized.

【惊蛰食疗方：带鱼春笋汤】

材料：带鱼 500g，春笋 100g，咸肉 130g，黑木耳 16g，黄酒 10g，红椒 1/2 只，大葱 1 根，生姜 4 片，蒜 1/2 个，盐适量。

做法：带鱼洗净，切成 6cm 的长条状；咸肉清洗，切薄片，黑木耳用温水泡发后清洗干净，大葱斜切 3cm 的小段；春笋去壳清洗后斜切成片。铁锅预热后放油，下带鱼块文火煎至两面微黄铲起；另起油锅，放葱、蒜、姜片微煸成金黄色，倒入咸肉煸炒后加黄酒；加入煎好的带鱼，以及春笋、黑木耳和红椒；倒入热水，武火烧开后转文火煮 20 分钟左右，汤色呈奶白后下盐调味即可。

功效：益气健脾。

适宜人群：一般人群均可食用。尤其适合久病体虚、营养不良所致的头晕者。

Diet therapy: Spring Bamboo Shoots and Ribbonfish Soup

Ingredients: Ribbonfish 500g, spring bamboo shoots 100g, salt meat 130g, wood ear 16g, yellow rice wine 10g, half of a red pepper, one piece of leek, four slices of ginger, half of a clove of garlic, appropriate amount of salt.

Methods: Wash the ribbonfish and cut it into strips of 6 cm long. Wash the salt meat, and cut it into thin slices. Soak the wood ear in warm water and rinse the rehydrated wood ear. Cut the leek obliquely into small pieces of 3 cm long. Remove the shell of the bamboo shoots and cut them into slices obliquely after cleaning. Preheat the iron pan, add oil, and fry the ribbonfish with mild fire until both sides are yellowish. Prepare another pot with oil, add leek, garlic, ginger slices, and stir-fry them until they turn yellow, then add the salt meat and keep stir-frying. Add yellow rice wine, fried ribbonfish, spring bamboo shoots, wood ear and red pepper before pouring in hot water. Heat with strong fire and switch to mild fire for another 20 minutes after the soup boils. When the color of soup turns milky white, season the soup with salt and it is completed.

Actions: Benefiting qi and strengthening the spleen.

Indicated population: Everyone, especially those with dizziness due to prolonged diseases and malnutrition.

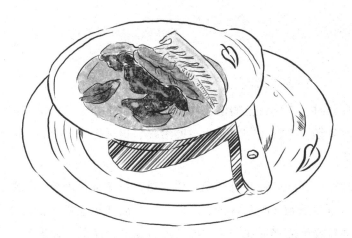

春分 Spring Equinox (Chunfen)

春分为每年公历 3 月 21 日前后，太阳黄经为 0°。春分以后，太阳直射位置更向北移，北半球开始昼长夜短。所以，春分是北半球春季的开始，我国大部分地区越冬作物进入生长阶段。

Each year around March 21st, the sun is exactly at the celestial longitude of 0°, which signifies the arrival of *Spring Equinox* (Chunfen). After *Spring Equinox*, daylight hours gradually increase as the sun continues to climb higher in the sky in the Northern Hemisphere. Therefore, *Spring Equinox* marks the beginning of spring of the Northern Hemisphere and the growth stage of overwintering crops in most area of China.

【春分养生误区】Misunderstandings of health nurturing

误区一：滋补过甚

春分时，人体胃肠的消化功能较差，也是呼吸道疾病和慢性疾病的高发期，滋补过甚，易生口腔溃疡、口干舌燥、手心脚心发热等病症。

预防：春分进补要有原则、要适量，不能盲目进补。注意五味调和，可以适当多吃富含糖、脂肪、蛋白质和维生素的食物补充能量，在饮食上适当增加苦味，如苦瓜、莴笋、芹菜、香椿等。

❶Excessive nourishing

In *Spring Equinox* there is decreased digestive function and high incidence of respiratory diseases and chronic diseases. Excessive nourishing can induce mouth ulcers, dry mouth, feverish feeling in the soles and palms, etc.

Prevention: Remember to nourish appropriately according to certain principles. The balanced combination of five flavors is emphasized. Foods that are rich in glucose, fat, proteins, and vitamins can be chosen for energy supplement. Food that is bitter in flavor can be added, such as bitter gourd, stem lettuce, celery, and Xiangchun (Chinese toon sprouts), etc.

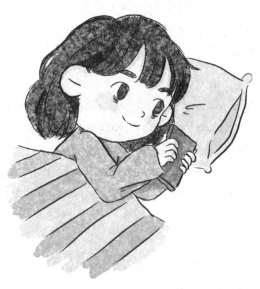

误区二：睡得太晚

春分过后昼长夜短，很多人 23 时后入睡，甚至熬夜，极易损伤肝脏，也易引发失眠。

预防：保证每天 6 ～ 8 小时的睡眠，同时还可按摩太阳穴、晒晒太阳、听听舒缓的音乐，有助于睡眠。

❷Sleeping too late

As the duration of daytime increases after *Spring Equinox*, many persons tend to sleep after 11 pm and even stay up, which will harm the liver and cause insomnia.

Prevention: Six-to-eight-hour sleep each day is essential. Besides, it is beneficial to sleep to massage the temple, take sunbath, and listen to slow music.

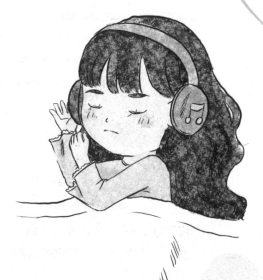

误区三：活动不当

所谓"三月不减肥，四月徒伤悲"，春分一到，越来越多的人开始加大活动量，但活动过度易导致关节损伤。

预防：建议活动时间控制在 1 小时内为佳，且活动地点应选择清晨空气清新之处。

❸ Excessive exercises

As *Spring Equinox* arrives, more and more people begin to increase the amount of exercises to lose weight, but excessive exercises can easily lead to joint injuries.

Prevention: It is suggested to exercise for no more than one hour each time in the morning, and the chosen place should be filled with fresh air.

误区四：穿得太少

春分"倒春寒"时常出现，衣着单薄的人不但容易感冒，也会增加心脑血管疾病发生的概率。

预防：上衣轻薄，裤子、鞋袜注意保暖，春分仍然需要适当"捂一捂"。

❹ Dressing too little

Cold snaps can occur often in *Spring Equinox*. Those who dress too little can easily catch colds, and the risk of cardiovascular and cerebro-vascular diseases is increased.

Prevention: Wear light and thin clothing in the upper body, while wear warm clothing in the lower part, including trousers, shoes, and sacks. Appropriate "covering-up" is still needed.

【春分食疗方：山药核桃羹】

材料：核桃仁 15g，山药 20g，冰糖少许。

做法：将核桃仁炒香，同山药共研成细粉；冰糖放入开水中溶化成汁；将适量水加入砂锅内，煮沸，将核桃仁与山药粉、冰糖汁加入，不断搅拌，待成糊状即可。

功效：健脾除湿，固肾止遗。

适宜人群：精神疲倦、全身困倦乏力、食欲不振、稀便，以及妇女白带夹红、淋沥不尽者等。

Diet therapy: Yam and Walnut Paste

Ingredients: Walnuts 15g, yam 20g, several cubes of rock sugar.

Methods: Stir-fry walnuts until fragrant, and grind them into fine powder together with yam. Dissolve the rock sugar in boiling water. Boil appropriate amount of water in the casserole, then add the powder and sugar juice and stir it into paste.

Actions: Strengthening the spleen to eliminate dampness, and securing the kidney to stop leakage.

Indicated population: Those with lassitude, lack of strength, poor appetite, loose stool, and women with prolonged leukorrhea combined with blood.

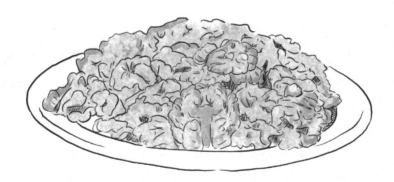

清明 Fresh Green (Qingming)

清明为每年公历 4 月 5 日前后，太阳黄经为 15°。此时气候清爽温暖，草木开始发新的枝芽，万物开始生长，农民忙于春耕。在清明节这一天，有家门口插杨柳枝条、郊外踏青及祭扫坟墓等习俗。

Fresh Green (Qingming) falls on around April 5th when the sun reaches the celestial longitude of 15°. The days are going to be warm and fresh (when not raining), and the vegetation turns green. While things begin to grow, peasants are still busy with spring plowing. There are various customs for Chinese people in *Fresh Green*, such as hanging willow branches, spring outing and tomb sweeping.

【清明时节重舒心】Keeping an peaceful mind

❶ 调控情绪

清明既是一个中医养生的重要节气，又是踏青扫墓、追悼先人、悲痛伤感的祭祀节日。有心脑血管疾病、血压偏高者，应注意不要劳累或伤心，扫墓时最好有亲人陪伴。

❶Regulating emotions

Fresh Green is an important solar term for health nurturing in traditional Chinese medicine (TCM). It is also a festival for tomb sweeping to pay respects to those who have died, which will inevitably arouse a mood of melancholy. Those with cardiovascular and cerebrovascular diseases should not be overstrained or too grieved, and should be accompanied when visit the graves.

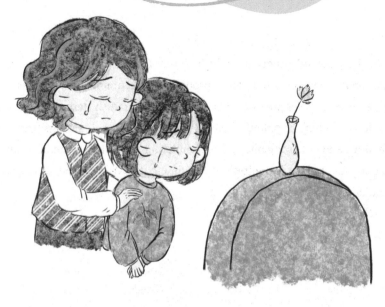

❷ "动" 不宜大

清明有踏青、放风筝、荡秋千等放松身心的习俗，踏青登山一定要量力而行，不要逞强好胜而一鼓作气地爬上去，以免发生意外。

❷ Avoiding strenuous activities

Fresh Green is a good time for relaxing activities like spring outing, kite flying and swing playing. When climbing the mountain for spring outing, remember to act according to your own strength, and avoid overloading yourself in case accidents happen.

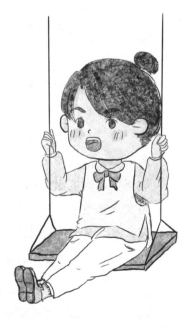

❸ 忌食 "生发"

清明多雨阴湿、乍暖还寒，饮食宜温，如韭菜、红薯、白菜、萝卜、芋头等时令蔬菜，不宜食用带鱼、黄鱼、鲳鱼、蚌肉、虾、螃蟹等海产类和竹笋、芥菜、南瓜、菠菜等蔬菜类发物，容易诱发旧疾，或加重现有疾病。

❸ Avoiding stimulating food

There is still lingering cold in *Fresh Green* in wet and rainy days. Seasonal foods that are warm in property are recommended, such as Chinese chives, sweet potatoes, Chinese cabbage, radish, taro, etc. Seafood such as ribbonfish, yellow croaker, butterfish, mussel, shrimp, and crab should be avoided together with stimulating vegetables such as bamboo shoots, leaf mustard, pumpkin, spinach, etc. to avoid relapse or aggravation of existing diseases.

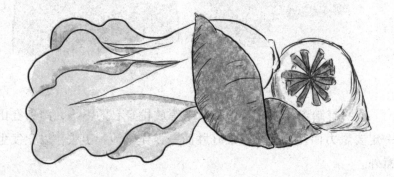

【清明食疗方：香酥山药】

材料：山药 500g，白砂糖 125g，淀粉 100g，植物油、米醋、味精等适量。

做法：山药洗净，用武火蒸熟，去皮，切成 3cm 长段，再一剖两半，拍扁待用。在锅中放植物油，待烧至七成热时，放山药，炸至黄色时取出。锅内留少许油，加炸好的山药、白糖、两勺水，用文火烧 5～6 分钟后，转用武火，加米醋、味精后，用淀粉勾芡，淋上熟油，装盘即成。

功效：健脾胃，补肺肾。

适宜人群：一般人群均可食用。尤其适合食欲不佳、容易疲倦、腹胀、腹泻等病症的机体虚弱者。

Ingredients: Henan yam 500g, white sugar 125g, starch 100g, appropriate amount of vegetable oil, rice vinegar, and MSG (monosodium glutamate).

Methods: Wash the yams and steam it with strong fire. Peel the yams and cut them into cylindrical discs of 3 cm long, then cut them in half and pat them flat. Pour vegetable oil into the pot, and preheat the oil to about 170℃. Add the yams and stir the chips till they have turned golden. Leave a little oil in the pot, add fried yam, white sugar and two spoons of water, and heat with mild fire for 5 to 6 minutes before switching to strong fire, then add rice vinegar and MSG. Thicken the yams with starch, and pour cooked oil before serving on a plate.

Actions: Strengthening the spleen and stomach, and nourishing the lung and kidney.

Indicated population: Everyone, especially those with weak constitution, manifesting as poor appetite, lack of strength, abdominal distension, and diarrhea.

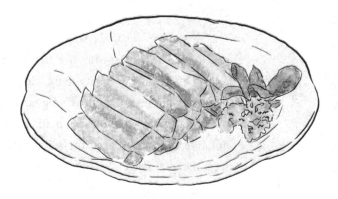

春季 SPRING

谷雨 Grain Rain (Guyu)

谷雨为每年公历 4 月 20 日前后，太阳黄经为 30°。谷雨就是雨水生五谷的意思。由于雨水滋润大地，五谷得以生长，谷雨就是"雨生百谷"，是春作物播种、出苗的季节。

Every year around April 20 when the sun reaches the celestial longitude of 30° comes *Grain Rain* (Guyu). Literally it means "rain for grain", which indicates that plentiful rainfall nourishes the crops. Therefore, it's the best time for sowing and sprouting of seeds.

【谷雨警惕风湿病复发】Be aware of rheumatism relapse

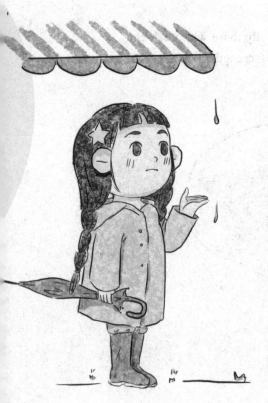

❶ 家居防潮

谷雨预示着雨季的到来，这时空气水分量大，要注意防潮。尤其是有风湿病患者，要注意不要久居潮湿之地，不要穿潮湿的衣服。

❶ Preventing dampness

Grain Rain denotes the forthcoming rains. Due to high humidity in the air, prevention of dampness should be emphasized. In particular, patients with rheumatism should not live in damp places for a long time or wear damp clothes.

❷ 注意保暖

谷雨意味着离夏天不远了，但早晚温差还是较大。所以，早晚外出时应注意保暖，避免吹风，多带一件稍厚的衣服，并注意关节部位的保暖，避免淋雨。

❷Keeping warm

Grain Rain, though signifying the approaching of summer, is still featured by marked temperature difference between morning and evening. When going out in the morning and evening, remember to keep yourself, especially the joints, warm; take a warm clothing along, and avoid wind and rain.

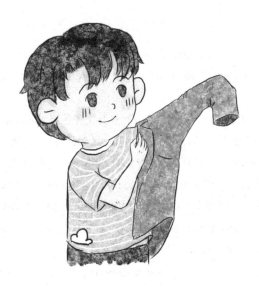

❸ 吃祛湿食物

在返潮天应多吃祛湿食物，如蘑菇、豆腐或老鸭等配成的汤，有祛湿排汗的作用。

❸Taking dampness-eliminating food

In the humid days, food that can eliminate dampness can be chosen, such as stewed old duck with mushroom and tofu, which can promote diaphoresis and remove dampness.

【谷雨食疗方：冬瓜海带荷叶排骨汤】

材料：带皮冬瓜 500～600g，干荷叶 5g，海带 50g，排骨 150g，生姜 3 片切丝，盐适量。

做法：排骨洗净氽烫，冬瓜带皮切块，干荷叶洗净放入棉织布袋中，其他材料洗干净备用；水煮沸后放入所有材料，武火煮10分钟，再转文火熬2.5小时，加入少许盐调味即可。

功效：清热除湿，消肿利尿。

适宜人群：胃口欠佳，肢体易疲倦，头晕头胀，关节、肌肉酸痛，小便量少者。

Diet therapy: Rib Soup with White Gourd, Kelp, and Lotus Leaves

Ingredients: White gourd (unpeeled) 500-600g, dry lotus leaves 5g, kelp 50g, ribs 15 g, 3 slices of ginger (shredded), appropriate amount of salt.

Methods: Blanch ribs in boiling water. Chop the unpeeled white gourd into small pieces. Wash the dry lotus leaves and put them into a cotton bag. Prepare a pot of boiling water and add all of the ingredients that has been washed. Boil with strong fire for ten minutes and then simmer the soup for another 2.5 hours before seasoning with salt.

Actions: Clearing heat and removing dampness, promoting urination and eliminating edema.

Indicated population: Those with poor appetite, lack of strength in the limbs, dizziness and distending sensation of the head, aching pain in the joints and muscles, as well as oliguria.

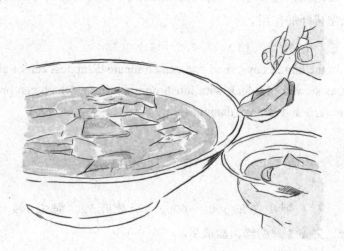

夏季 SUMMER

夏三月，起于立夏，止于立秋前。夏季分为立夏、小满、芒种、夏至、小暑、大暑六个节气。

Summer includes three months between *Beginning of Summer* (Lixia) and *Beginning of Autumn* (Liqiu), which can be divided into six solar terms: *Beginning of Summer*, *Lesser Fullness* (Xiaoman), *Grain in Ear* (Mangzhong), *Summer Solstice* (Xiazhi), *Lesser Heat* (Xiaoshu), and *Greater Heat* (Dashu).

夏季为四季之盛，日长夜短，内陆地区干燥酷热，沿海地区潮湿闷热，七月下旬和八月上旬常常是大雨和暴雨的集中期。

Summer is the season of the strongest yang qi with longer days and shorter nights. It is dry and hot in inland areas, while humid and sultry in coastal areas. There is also heavy rain in late July and early August.

夏季气候炎热应注意防晒。外出时衣着材质以轻、薄、柔软为佳，宜穿浅色服装，透气性、吸热性越好，越能有效地帮助人体散热。夏季居处开窗通风最好选择晚上 8 时到次日 8 时。

Sun protection should be emphasized in hot summer. When going out, you should choose light thin and soft clothing of light color which can well absorb the heat and allows your skin to breathe freely as it can help the body to dissipate heat more effectively. Besides, it is better to open windows from 8 pm to 8 am of the next day.

宜：夏季饮食应以健脾、祛暑化湿为主，可选择山药、枸杞子、鸭肉、黑豆等清淡食物。

Recommended: Light food that can strengthen the spleen, expel summer-heat and eliminate dampness can be chosen, such as yam, Chinese wolfberry, duck meat, and black soybean.

不宜：夏季不宜食用过多的冷冻食物，体质虚寒者不宜食用西瓜、香瓜、芒果等寒性水果，体质过敏者不宜食用芒果和鱼等。

Not recommended: Too much frozen food. Fruits that are cold in property, such as watermelon, muskmelon, and mango are not suitable for those with deficiency-cold constitution. Those prone to allergies should avoid mango and fish.

饮食

【首选蔬菜：黄瓜】Preferred vegetable: cucumber

夏季天气炎热，对人体最重要的影响是暑湿。暑湿侵入人体后会导致毛孔张开、过多出汗，引起肠胃功能失调，这时可多食用黄瓜。黄瓜具有生津止渴、除烦解暑、清热利水、排毒通便的作用。肝病、心血管疾病、肠胃疾病及高血压患者不宜过多食用。

Summer-heat dampness affects the body mostly in hot summer. The invasion of summer-heat dampness will lead to opening of pores that will further induce excessive sweeting. Besides, it can also influence the function the spleen and stomach. Cucumber is recommended in summer as it can promote fluid production to quench thirst, eliminate vexation and summer-heat, clear heat and promote urination, expel pathogen and promote defecation. However, those with liver diseases, cardiovascular diseases, digestive diseases, and hypertension shouldn't eat too much cucumber.

【首选鱼类：鲤鱼】Preferred fish: carp

夏初的鲤鱼正值产卵季，这时的鲤鱼富含优质蛋白、矿物质和维生素，极易被消化吸收。夏季气候温热潮湿，适当喝些鲤鱼汤，有助于祛湿开胃、利水消肿。儿童、孕妇、老年人等各类人群皆适宜食用，但荨麻疹、皮肤湿疹、支气管哮喘等患者慎食。

In the early summer carp spawn. At this time, the carp is rich in high-quality protein, minerals and vitamins, which are easily digested and absorbed. Carp soup is recommended for everyone, especially children, pregnant women, and the elderly in such a humid and sultry summer. It can dispel dampness to increase the appetite, promoting diuresis and edema. However, the soup is not recommended for patients with urticaria, eczema, and bronchial asthma.

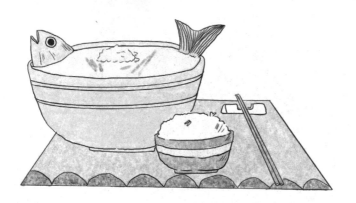

【首选菌类：木耳】Preferred fungus: wood ear

木耳味甘、性平，具有润肺等功效，夏季多吃点黑木耳，既有利于排毒通便，又可增加食欲。木耳适合心脑血管疾病、结石症等患者食用，但有出血性疾病、腹泻者及孕妇应少食。

With sweet flavor and balanced property, wood ear is capable of nourishing the lung. It is recommended in summer as it can help detoxify the body and promote defecation, and increase the appetite. It is suitable for those with cardiovascular and cerebrovascular diseases or lithiasis. However, the dosage should be decreased in pregnant women and those with hemorrhagic diseases, and diarrhea.

【首选肉类：鸭肉】Preferred meat: duck meat

鸭肉富含人体在夏季急需的蛋白质等营养物质，适合体质虚弱、食欲不佳、大便干燥和水肿者食用。但慢性肠炎等患者应少食。

Due to high content of proteins which is needed in summer, duck meat is suitable for those with weak constitution, poor appetite, dry stool, and edema. However, those with chronic enteritis should eat less duck meat.

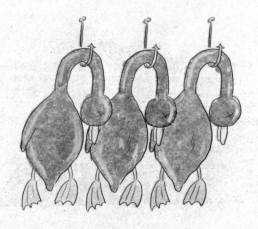

【首选谷类：薏仁】Preferred grain: pearl barley

薏仁性味甘淡微寒，含有维生素 B1 和多种氨基酸，有利水消肿、健脾、清热等功效。孕妇、消化不良者不宜食用。

Pearl barley, sweet and bland in flavor and slightly cold in property, contains vitamin B1, and various amino acids. It can promote urination to eliminate edema, strengthen the spleen and clear heat. However, it is not recommended for pregnant women and those with dyspepsia.

【首选粥类：绿豆粥】
Preferred porridge: Mung Bean Porridge

绿豆粥具有清热解毒、消暑等作用，是夏季人们较喜欢的消暑粥类。但寒凉体质的人，如四肢冰凉乏力、腹泻便稀等不宜食用；老年人、儿童及体质虚弱者也不宜过多食用。

Mung Bean Porridge is favored in summer as it can cleat heat and detoxify the body, and eliminate summer-heat. However, it is not recommended for those with deficiency-cold constitution with symptoms of cold and weak limbs, diarrhea or loose stool. The dosage should be decreased in the elderly, children and those with deficient constitution.

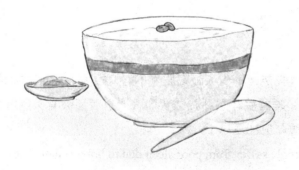

【首选饮品：酸梅汤】
Preferred drink: Sour Plum Drink

酸梅汤由乌梅、山楂、桂花、甘草、冰糖组成，有止渴、安神的功效，对于夏季而言是消暑解渴的饮品之选，老少皆宜，但有胃病者不宜多饮。

Sour Plum Drink is made from smoked plum, hawthorn fruit, Osmanthus blossoms, liquorice, and rock sugar. It can quench thirst and relax the mind and is thus favored by the old and the young in summer. However, those with stomach diseases shouldn't drink too much.

【首选瓜类：西瓜】Preferred melon: watermelon

西瓜具有清热、解暑、止渴等功效，夏天出汗多，适当吃些西瓜，能补足丢失的水分。肾功能不全、产妇及糖尿病患者不宜食用。

Watermelon is capable of clearing heat, eliminating summer-heat, and quenching thirst. Appropriate amount of watermelon can help supplement moisture loss due to profuse sweating in summer. It is not recommended for women after delivery or those with kidney failure or diabetes.

睡眠

夏季天气炎热，不少人睡眠质量不好，很多人喜欢睡觉时开着风扇、空调，睡醒后却感到腰酸背痛，严重者还会有头痛等症状。因此，夏季睡眠应注意以下几点。

Many people suffer from poor sleep due to hot weather. They like to sleep with the fan or air conditioner on. On the next day, they might feel backache and even headache and other symptoms. Pay attention to the following tips for sleep in summer.

【忌在空调通风口睡觉】
Avoiding facing the vent of air conditioner

夏季天气炎热，很多人喜欢在空调通风口睡觉，容易引起感冒、头痛等症状，严重者甚至出现面瘫，所以最好避免在通风口处睡觉，同时也不宜选择过堂风口之处。

Many people like to sleep toward the vent of air conditioner in hot summer. However, this might lead to contraction of colds, headache, and even facial paralysis. It is suggested to avoid facing the vent or draught when sleep.

【忌袒胸露腹睡觉】Avoiding exposing the belly

袒胸露腹睡觉容易受凉，因此，无论天气多热，都要在胸腹部盖上一层薄被子或毯子，以免受凉后导致腹痛、腹泻。

Cold might invade the body when sleeping with the belly exposed. Therefore, you should cover your belly with a thin blanket or quilt anyhow in case abdominal pain and diarrhea occur after contraction of cold.

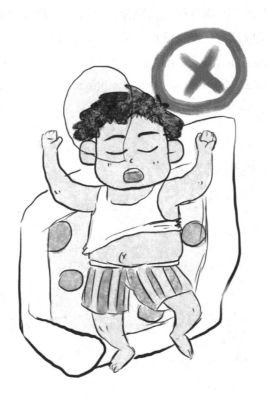

【忌用冷水擦凉席】
Avoiding mopping mat with cold water

凉席本身并不干燥，如再用冷水擦拭，将会增加床的湿度，使床成为各类霉菌及细菌的滋生地。建议使用热水擦拭凉席，擦拭后用电风扇将其吹干。

The dry summer sleeping mat will absorb moisture if being mopped with cold water, which will make the bed an ideal breeding ground for bacteria and moulds. It is, therefore, suggested to mop the mat with hot water and then dry it with a fan.

【忌入睡后开空调、电风扇】
Avoiding sleeping with air conditioner or fan on

入睡后人体血液循环往往会减慢，抵抗力也相对较弱，长时间开着空调或风扇睡觉，极易受凉，从而引发感冒。

During sleep, blood circulation of the body will be slowed and immunity decreased. Sleeping with air conditioner or fan on will make it much easier to catch colds.

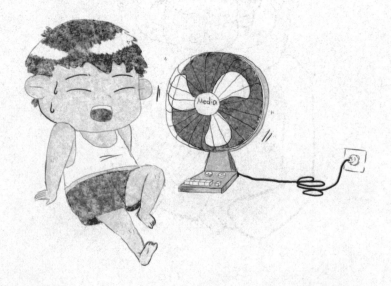

活动

夏季天气日渐炎热，贸然进行不恰当的活动，反而适得其反。所以，入夏后宜选择体能消耗少、技术要求低、时间消耗适宜的活动。具体推荐以下几项活动。

Inappropriate exercises without consideration will, on the contrary, do harm to the body in such hot weather. It is suggested to do exercises that take proper time and require less strength and skills. The following exercises are recommended.

【散步】Strolling

夏季散步应注意选择在树荫下或者有风的河边、海边或公园的林荫道，时间控制在 1 小时内。此法适宜中老年人和体质稍弱者，但高血压患者早晨血压最高，傍晚相对稳定，建议此类人群选择晚饭后散步；糖尿病患者不能饿肚子散步，易导致低血糖；冠心病患者散步速度要慢，以免心律失常。

It is necessary to stroll under shade or along the river where there is breeze for no more than one hour. It is suitable for the elderly and the infirm. Due to high blood pressure in the morning, those with hypertension should stroll after supper when the blood pressure is relatively stable. Those with diabetes shouldn't walk on an empty stomach, because it can lead to hypoglycemia. Those with coronary heart disease should walk slowly to avoid arrhythmia.

【瑜伽】Yoga

瑜伽四季皆宜，夏季练习瑜伽更有益身心，缓解因天气炎热而带来的焦虑，练习瑜伽应选择通风、凉爽之地，时间控制在45 ～ 60分钟。有脊椎病、腰椎间盘突出、骨关节病、骨性关节炎等疾病者，练习瑜伽时应尤其慎重，练习前应当咨询专科医师。

Yoga is suitable in the four seasons, especially in summer. It is beneficial to both the body and mind, and can relieve anxiety in the hot weather. Yoga should be practiced in a ventilated and cool place for 45 to 60 minutes. Those with spondylosis, lumbar herniated disc, osteoarthritis and other diseases should be especially careful when practicing yoga, and should consult a specialist before practicing.

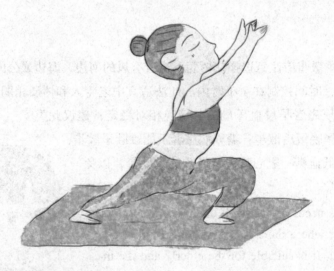

【游泳】Swimming

夏季是游泳的最佳季节，游泳具有减肥、降低胆固醇、增强心血管功能等作用。游泳消耗体能较大，时间应控制在2小时内。患有心脏病、糖尿病、肺病等疾病者应在听取医生建议后方可游泳，以免发生意外。

Summer is the best season for swimming. It can help reduce weight, decrease the level of cholesterol and enhance cardiovascular function. The time should be no more than two hours as swimming consumes a lot of energy. Patients suffering from heart disease, diabetes and lung diseases should swim after consulting the doctors so as to avoid accidents.

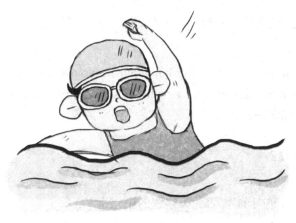

【室内羽毛球】Indoor badminton

室内羽毛球因无日晒烦恼，而成了夏季活动的理想选择之一。

打羽毛球不仅强身健体、减肥塑身、预防颈椎病，还可促进新陈代谢，使体内毒素随汗排出。活动时间可根据自身情况而定，青少年以 40 ～ 50 分钟为宜，老年人和体弱者以 20 ～ 30 分钟为宜。患有心血管疾病者，剧烈运动会加重病情。

Without exposure to the sun, indoor badminton is an ideal choice in summer.

It can not only strengthen the body, lose weight and prevent cervical spondylosis, but also promote metabolism and excrete toxins with sweat. The time of activity can be adjusted according to your own situation, 40-50 minutes for teenagers, 20-30 minutes for the elderly and the frail. Patients with cardiovascular disease should avoid this exercise, as strenuous exercise will aggravate the disease.

穴位养生

夏季天气炎热，此时人体心气旺盛，出汗多，因此，养心尤为重要。

Heart qi is most strong in hot summer. Nourishing the heart is of great importance due to large amount of sweat which is believed to be the fluid of the heart.

膻中穴

【位置】位于前胸两乳头连线的中点上。

【功效】按摩膻中穴，对心、肺、胃之功能有调节作用。

【方法】先用大拇指按揉膻中穴3分钟，由轻到重，以能承受为度，或艾炷灸膻中穴 5～7 壮，或艾条灸 10～20 分钟。按摩膻中穴时配合按摩内关穴（见下文）效果会更好。

Danzhong (CV 17)

Location: At the midpoint between the nipples.

Actions: Regulating the function of the heart, lung, and stomach.

Methods: Massage the acupoint with thumb for 3 minutes, and gradually increase pressure as much as you can tolerate. At the same time, the combination of acupressure on Neiguan (PC 6) can boost the effects. What's more, moxibustion with 5 to 7 moxa cones or with moxa

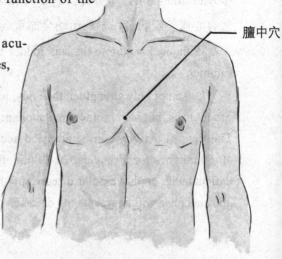

膻中穴

stick for 10 to 20 minutes can also be chosen.

至阳穴

【位置】位于背部第七、八胸椎棘突之间，约与肩胛骨下角相平。

【功效】心脏不适、胸口发紧时，可按摩至阳穴，以利于心脏供血。

【方法】可取小型刮痧板，用右手食指拇指夹持，以刮痧板的横缘抵住至阳穴，予以重压，以局部有酸胀感为度，5 ～ 10 分钟为宜。

Zhiyang (GV 9)

Location: Between the seventh and eighth spinous process of thoracic vertebra, at the level of inferior angle of the scapula.

Actions: Promoting blood supply to the heart when pressed, which can be used for discomfort and tightness in the chest.

Methods: Hold small-sized scraping tool with right thumb and index finger, press the transverse edge against the acupoint. Increase pressure until there is soreness and distending sensation, then hold it for 5-10 minutes.

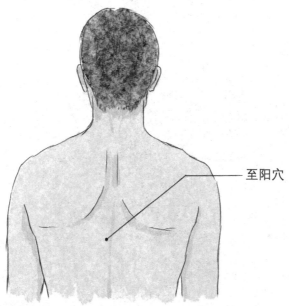

至阳穴

内关穴

【位置】位于手掌面关节横纹的中央，往上约三指宽的中央凹陷处。

【功效】按摩内关穴，能缓解心悸、胸闷、胸痛，也可缓解失眠。

【方法】心悸或胸闷时，按压内关穴，以症状缓解为度，也可于每日睡前按压双侧内关穴 100 次，以帮助入睡。

Neiguan (PC 6)

Location: In the depression between two tendons, about three fingers width above the transverse crease of the wrist.

Actions: Relieving palpitations, chest tightness and pain, as well as insomnia.

Methods: Press the acupoints for palpitations and chest tightness until you feel relieved. The acupoints on both sides can be pressed for 100 times each night to help you fall asleep.

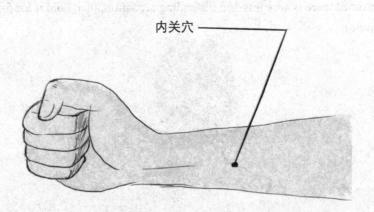

内关穴

立夏 Beginning of Summer (Lixia)

立夏为每年公历 5 月 6 日前后，太阳黄经为 45°。立夏是夏季的开始，万物旺盛。人们习惯上把立夏当作气温显著升高、炎暑将临、雷雨增多、农作物进入生长旺季的一个重要节气。

Each year around May 6th, when the sun reaches the celestial longitude of 45°, it marks the arrival of *Beginning of Summer* (Lixia), a solar term signifying the advent of hot summer and the growing season. It is believed that the solar term welcomes the markedly increase of heat and thunderstorms, as well as the rapid growing season of crops.

【立夏养生重养心】 Nourishing the heart

闭目养神其实也是在养心，所以，立夏除了午睡外，还可通过静坐、梳头养心。

Closing eyes for refreshing the mind is also a way to nourish the heart. In addition to taking a nap after lunch, the heart can also be nourished through combing the hair and meditation while sitting quietly.

❶ 静坐

每天上午 11 时至下午 1 时，让心脏休息一下是很养心的。如果没有条件午睡，可选择在办公室，或机场、车站等有座椅处静坐 3 分钟，以达到养心的目的。

❶ Meditation while sitting quietly

It is beneficial to the body to rest the heart from 11 am to 1 pm when heart qi is exuberant. If it is inconvenient to take a nap, you can choose meditation while sitting

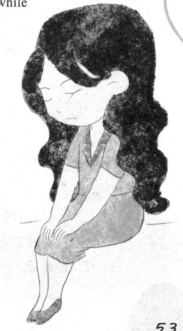

quietly where there are seats for the purpose of nourishing the heart.

❷ 梳头

梳头可以刺激头部的穴位，可疏通经络、调节神经功能，还能预防失眠、眩晕、心悸等。可每天用手指梳头 3～5 次，每次不少于 3 分钟或 5 分钟，晚上睡前可再做 3 次。

❷ Combing the hair

Through combing the hair, acupoints on the head are stimulated, which can dredge the meridians and collaterals and regulate nervous function, thus preventing insomnia, dizziness and palpitations. You can comb the hair with your hands for no less than 3 or 5 minutes each time, 3 to 5 times a day. It is also suggested to repeat such action three times before sleep.

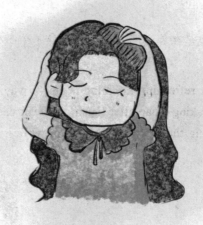

【立夏食疗方：丝瓜粥】

材料：丝瓜 100g，粳米 200～300g，盐、味精等调味品适量。

做法：将丝瓜去皮后切成小块待用。将粳米熬成粥，起锅前，放入切块的丝瓜，再煮开几分钟，加入适量调味品即可。

功效：清暑化痰。

适宜人群：一般人群均可食用。尤其适合口干、咳嗽咳痰、产后乳汁不通者。

Diet therapy: Sponge Gourd Porridge

Ingredients: Sponge gourd 100g, japonica rice 200-300g, appropriate amount of salt and MSG.

Methods: Peel and cut the sponge gourd into small pieces. Boil the japonica rice, then add the chopped sponge gourd, and boil for several minutes before seasoning.

Actions: Clearing summer-heat and eliminating phlegm.

Indicated population: Everyone, especially those with dry mouth, cough with phlegm, and inhibited lactation after delivery.

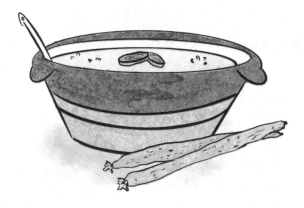

小满 Lesser Fullness (Xiaoman)

小满为每年公历 5 月 21 日前后，太阳黄经为 60°。从小满开始，大麦、冬小麦等夏收作物已经结果，但尚未成熟，故称小满。小满后，北方各地的小麦即将成熟，而黄淮流域的冬小麦将开镰收割。

Lesser Fullness (Xiaoman) falls around May 21st when the sun reaches the celestial longitude of 60°. Lesser Fullness denotes that summer crops such as barley and winter wheat have started to plump, but have not yet matured. After Lesser Fullness, wheat in the northern area is about to mature, while peasants from the Yellow and Huai Valleys are preparing harvest of winter wheat.

【 小满时节"健脾祛湿" 】During the Xiaoman season

❶ 宜健脾祛湿

小满后雨水渐多，人体的脾易受湿邪影响，这时饮食调理应注意健脾祛湿，以清爽清淡的素食为主，可多食赤小豆、薏仁、绿豆、冬瓜、山药、鲫鱼、酸梅汤、萝卜子等。

❶Strengthening the spleen and eliminating dampness

There is increased rainfall after Lesser Fullness, which tends to make the spleen subject to "damp pathogen". Fresh and light diet is recommended to invigorate the spleen and remove dampness, such as red bean, pearl barley, mung bean, white gourd, yam, crucian carp, Sour Plum Drink, radish seed, etc.

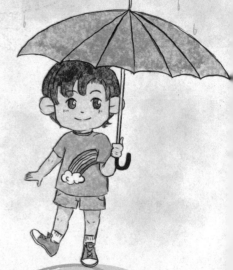

❷ 按揉足三里穴

小满雨水较多，此时养生的重点即祛湿，按摩足三里穴有利于人体水分的运行和排泄，具有防治疾病、强身健体的作用。用拇指着力于足三里穴，垂直用力，以酸胀为度，如此每天反复操作5～10次即可。

❷Massaging Zusanli (ST 36)

Emphasis should be placed on eliminating dampness when it comes to health nurturing in Lesser Fullness where there is plentiful rainfall. Massaging Zusanli (ST 36) can promote the transportation and metabolism of water, thus helping to prevent and treat certain diseases and build the body. Press the acupoints with your thumb and apply pressure vertical to the leg until there is soreness and distending sensation, which should be repeated five to ten times each day.

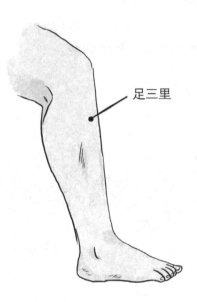

足三里

【小满食疗方：薏仁红绿豆浆】

材料：绿豆 20g，红豆 20g，薏仁 30g。

做法：绿豆、红豆、薏仁分别淘洗干净，用清水浸泡 5 小时至软；将泡好的绿豆、红豆、薏仁一同倒入全自动豆浆机中，加入适量水做成豆浆食用。

功效：健脾利湿，清热解毒。

适宜人群：口苦口渴、食欲不佳、小便黄赤，以及阴囊湿痒者。

Diet therapy: Soy Milk of Pearl Barley, Mung Bean and Red Bean

Ingredients: Mung beans 20 g, red beans 20 g, pearl barley 30 g.

Methods: Rinse the prepared ingredients and soak them for five hours until they turn soft. Put the soaked ingredients into automatic soy-milk machine and add appropriate amount of water.

Actions: Strengthening the spleen and eliminating dampness, clearing heat and detoxifying the body.

Indicated population: Those with bitter taste in the mouth, thirst, poor appetite, dark urine, and itchy groin.

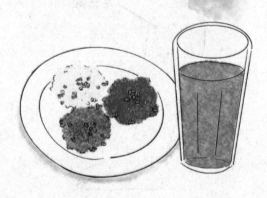

芒种 Grain in Ear (Mangzhong)

芒种为每年公历 6 月 6 日前后，太阳黄经为 75°。芒种即表明小麦等有芒作物成熟。芒种前后，我国长江中下游地区雨量增多、气温升高，进入连绵阴雨的梅雨季节。

Every year around June 6th Grain in Ear (Mangzhong) arrives as the sun reaches the celestial longitude of 75°. It marks the maturation of wheat and other crops. *Grain in Ear* usually kicks off a period of abundant rainfall, increased temperature and "plum rain" season in the middle-lower Yangtze River region.

【芒种重"三防"】Prevention of three diseases

❶ 防湿疹

芒种雨水逐渐增多，尤其南方空气湿度大，易生湿疹。凡急性发作的湿疹其发病原因不外湿、热、毒三种。所以，芒种时应不吃辛辣刺激、油炸类食物，不饮浓茶、咖啡，杜绝熬夜。

❶Preventing eczema

As rainfall increases gradually in Grain in Ear, the air humidity is especially high in the south, which might induce eczema. The causes of acute onset of eczema include dampness, heat, and toxin. Accordingly, you should avoid spicy and stimulating food, fried food, strong tea and coffee, as well as staying up.

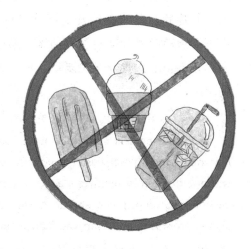

❷ 防伤脾

芒种天气较热，人们为了追求凉爽而过度吃生冷食物等，极易伤脾。此时应吃扁豆、胡萝卜、南瓜等温性食物，且少量食用冷饮。

❷Preventing damaging the spleen

Hot weather of Grain in Ear means it is more palatable eat cold and raw food, which, however, will easily cause damage to the spleen. Instead, food that are warm in property, such as lentil, carrot, and pumpkin can be chosen, and the intake of cold drinks should be decreased.

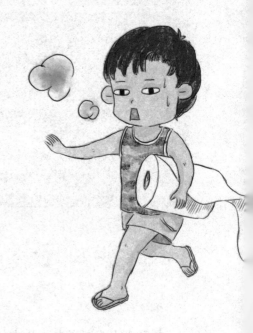

❸ 防热伤风

芒种后雨水渐多，暑热夹杂，易患热伤风。热伤风的常见症状为流涕、鼻塞、打喷嚏、发热、头痛等，有的患者还会出现呕吐、腹泻等症状。此时在饮食上可饮绿豆汤、金银花露、菊花茶、芦根茶以清热解暑。同时忌食油腻、酸腥、麻辣的食物。慎用补品，发热时不要吃人参及冬虫夏草、鹿茸等温性补品，也不要吃羊肉、狗肉。

❸Preventing contraction of warm-natured cold

Summer-heat is combined with increased rainfall after *Grain in Ear*, rendering it much easier to contract cold that is warm in nature. The warm-natured cold manifests as symptoms of running nose, nasal congestion, sneezing, fever, and headache, and in some cases, there might also be vomiting and diarrhea. Those capable of clearing summer-heat can be taken, such as Mung Bean Soup, Honeysuckle Tea, Chrysanthemum Tea, Reed Rhizome (Lugen) Tea. At the same time, avoid greasy, sour, raw or spicy food. Tonics should be used with caution. When there is fever, avoid those warm in property, such as tonics like ginseng, Chinese caterpillar fungus, deer velvet, as well as mutton and dog meat.

【芒种食疗方：鲜藕蛋羹】

材料：鲜藕 500g，鸡蛋 2 个，猪油少许，盐等调味品适量。

做法：将鸡蛋打入碗内调匀，将鲜藕榨成汁，将鸡蛋液倒入鲜藕汁中，加入少许猪油、盐等调料味品，最后将盛有鲜藕鸡蛋汁的碗放在蒸笼上，武火蒸 10 分钟即可。

功效：滋阴补血，健脾生津。

适宜人群：体虚易出虚汗、手心脚心等潮热者，以及产后体虚者。

Diet therapy: Steamed Egg Custard with Fresh Lotus Root Juice

Ingredients: Fresh lotus root 500g, 2 eggs, little lard, appropriate amount of seasoning, such as salt.

Methods: Whisk the eggs in a bowl and pour it into the prepared juice of fresh lotus root, add little lard, and salt before putting it on a steamer, then boil it with strong fire for ten minutes.

Actions: Nourishing yin and blood, strengthening the spleen and promoting fluid production.

Indicated population: Those with weak constitution manifesting as sweating, tidal fever in the palms and soles or weak women after delivery.

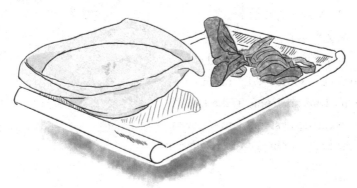

夏至 Summer Solstice (Xiazhi)

夏至为每年公历 6 月 21 日前后，太阳黄经为 90°。这一天是北半球白昼最长、黑夜最短的一天，从夏至起，进入炎热季节，大地万物在此时生长最旺盛。过了夏至，太阳逐渐向南移动，北半球白昼缩短，黑夜加长。

Summer Solstice (Xiazhi) generally occurs around June 21st when the sun reaches the celestial longitude of 90°. This solar term marks the longest daytime in the North Hemisphere, after which the sun gradually moves towards the South Hemisphere, thus decreasing the daytime and increasing the nighttime. Summer Solstice welcomes hot season when all things are experience the most vigorous growth.

【夏至重养生】Highlighting health nurturing

❶ 睡"子午觉"

"子"是指子时，即夜间 23 时至凌晨 1 时；"午"是指午时，即 11 ～ 13 时。在子午时间段内，机体各系统和器官处于需要调节、休整的状态，睡眠效果最佳，有缓解身体疲惫的作用。

❶ "Zi Wu (midday and midnight)" sleep

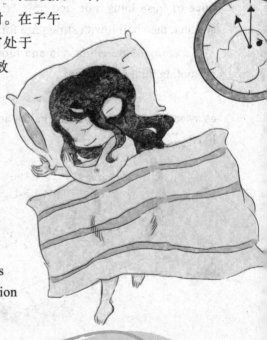

"Zi", refers to the period from 11 pm to 1 am of the next day, while "Wu" ranges from 11 am to 1 pm. In the two periods, the systems and organs in the body are in need of regulation and rest. And sleep at this time is often of high quality, which can relieve fatigue.

❷ 多吃"苦味"

人体肠胃受到炎热天气的刺激，消化功能相对较弱，饮食应以清淡为主。但夏至还要多吃有"苦"味的食物，如苦瓜、莲子心等，有助于清热、祛燥湿、止痒。但苦味的食物大多性寒，体弱者不宜多吃。

❷Increasing intake of bitter-flavored food

The hot weather tends to affect the digestive function. A light diet is therefore recommended. At the same time, food that is bitter in flavor can be taken such as bitter gourd, lotus plumule, etc., which can clear heat, eliminate dampness, and relieve itch. However, as most bitter-flavored food is cold in property, those with weak constitution should decrease the intake.

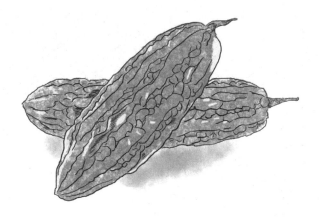

【 夏至食疗方：薏仁绿豆粥 】

材料：薏仁 200g，绿豆 100g，小米适量。

做法：薏仁在煮之前以温水浸泡 2 ～ 3 小时，绿豆最好也浸泡 1 ～ 2 小时，然后加入同等分量小米煮粥即可。

功效：健脾化湿，清热解暑。

适宜人群：暑热天气之胸闷、烦躁不安、口渴者，也适用于腹泻、水肿、小便不畅，以及四肢肌肉、关节紧张、僵硬者。

Diet therapy: Porridge of Pearl Barley and Mung Bean

Ingredients: Pear barley 200g, mung bean 100g, and appropriate amount of millet.

Methods: Soak the pearl barley for two to three hours in warm water, and the mung bean for one to two hours. Boil the prepared pearl barley and mung bean with equal amount of millet.

Actions: Strengthening the spleen and transforming dampness, clearing summer-heat.

Indicated population: Those with chest tightness, vexation, and thirst in hot weather, and those with diarrhea, edema, inhibited urination, and stiff and tight muscles and joints of the limbs.

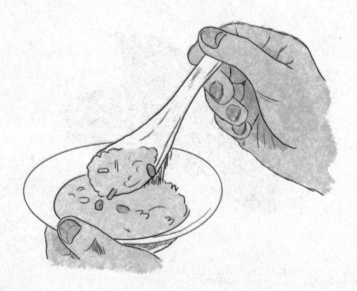

小暑 Lesser Heat (Xiaoshu)

小暑为每年公历 7 月 7 日前后，太阳黄经为 105°。此时，天气已接近炎热，但未到最热之时，故称为小暑。

With *Lesser Heat* (Xiaoshu) coming around July 7th as the sun reaches the celestial longitude of 105°, the summer heat wave arrives. However, just as the name--Lesser Heat indicates, the hottest days are yet to come.

【小暑养生重敷贴】Acupoint application

"冬病夏治"是我国传统中医药疗法中的特色疗法，是指对于一些在冬季易发生或加重的疾病，在夏季给予针对性的治疗，以提高机体的抗病能力。冬病夏治中最常用的方法为中药穴位敷贴，中药穴位敷贴应注意以下几点。

"Treating winter diseases in summer" is a unique principle of TCM. It refers to prescribe targeted therapy to enhance immunity against the diseases which easily occur or worsen in winter. The most frequently used therapeutic method is acupoint application with Chinese herbal medicine. The following tips should be observed.

❶ 适宜敷贴的疾病

心脑血管系统疾病：头痛、高血压、冠心病、心绞痛等。

消化系统疾病：慢性胃炎、消化性溃疡、胃肠功能紊乱、慢性结肠炎、慢性腹泻、消化不良等。

呼吸系统疾病：慢性支气管炎、肺气肿、肺源性心脏病、支气管哮喘、慢性阻塞性肺疾病等。

女性生殖系统疾病：月经不调、痛经、慢性盆腔炎等。

过敏性疾病：变应性鼻炎、慢性变应性咽炎、慢性荨麻疹、过敏性鼻炎等。

骨关节疾病：颈椎病、肩周炎、慢性腰肌劳损、四肢关节炎等。

❶Indicated population

Cardiovascular and cerebrovascular diseases: headache, hypertension, coronary heart disease, angina pectoris, etc.

Digestive diseases: chronic gastritis, peptic ulcer, gastrointestinal dysfunction, chronic colitis, chronic diarrhea, dyspepsia, etc.

Respiratory diseases: chronic bronchitis, emphysema, pulmonary heart disease, bronchial asthma, chronic obstructive pulmonary disease, etc.

Female reproductive system diseases: irregular menstruation, dysmenorrhea, chronic pelvic inflammatory disease, etc.

Allergic diseases: allergic rhinitis, chronic allergic pharyngitis, chronic urticaria, etc.

Bone and joint diseases: cervical spondylosis, frozen shoulder, chronic lumbar muscle strain, arthritis of the limbs, etc.

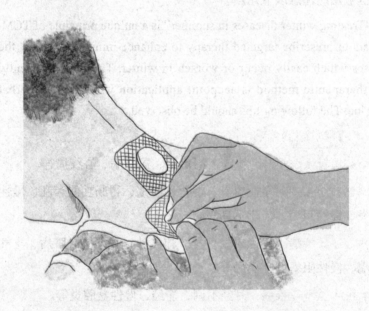

❷ 敷贴时间

在每年小暑后三伏天 [1] 当天敷贴，每 10 天贴 1 次。根据个人体质或对经络和穴位的敏感度不同而时间各异，儿童每次 0.5 ～ 1 小时，成人 2 ～ 4 小时。

❷ Time and duration

It should be carried out on the first day of the three ten-day periods of the hot season[1] after Lesser Heat, once every ten days. The duration varies from individuals according to their constitutions and sensitivity of acupoints to medicines. For the children, it should be 0.5 to 1 hour; while for the adults, it should be 2 to 4 hours.

[1] 三伏天：指一年内气温最高、湿度最大的时候，分为初伏、中伏和末伏，其中初伏和末伏均固定为 10 天，中伏有的年份 10 天，有的年份 20 天。伏期开始称入伏或交伏，伏期结束称出伏。

[1] Three ten-day periods of the hot season: Together they compose of the days of the highest temperature and humidity in a year. They include the beginning, the middle and the ending periods, among which the beginning and ending periods are ten days, while the middle period might include twenty days in some cases. The beginning of a period is called "entering or alternating", while the ending of a period is called "exiting".

❸ 禁忌人群及注意事项

孕妇、1 岁以下儿童、敷贴局部皮肤有损者不宜敷贴，正在发热者也不宜敷贴。

❸ Contraindicated in

pregnant women, children under one year old, and those with fever or skin lesions in corresponding acupoints.

敷贴后禁忌：忌食生冷、辛辣、油腻、海鲜等食物，同时敷贴当天最好不要洗澡，且避免风扇直吹或在温度过低的空调房间久待。

Contraindications after acupoint application: Avoid raw, cold, spicy, and greasy food, as well as seafood. On the exact day after appli-

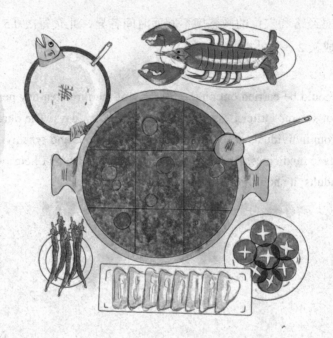

cation, do not take a bath, expose yourself directly to the fan, or stay too long in a room of low temperature with air conditioner on.

敷贴后护理：敷贴后，部分患者局部可能出现麻木、温、热、痒、针刺、疼痛等感觉，属于药物吸收的正常反应。如果难以忍受，须及时取下药物，并用清水冲洗局部。如局部出现水泡属正常现象，轻者可自抹万花油，若水泡溃破可自行涂紫药水，结痂后待自然去痂，注意防感染。若局部反应严重者，应及时到医院处理。

Management after acupoint application: It is normal if some patients present with local numbness, heat sensation, itch, pricking sensation, pain and other feelings in the absorption of medicines. When it is intolerable, take the medicines off in time and wash the area with clean water. There might also be blisters in the area. For mild condition, Wanhua Oil can be applied. If blisters burst, apply gentian violet and wait until the scab is removed naturally. During this time, attention should be placed on infection prevention. For severe cases, go to the hospital as soon as possible.

【小暑食疗方：莲子百合煨猪肉】

材料：莲子 50g，百合 50g，猪肉 200g，盐、葱、姜适量。

做法：将猪肉切成小块，把莲子、百合放入锅内加水，再加入盐、葱、姜，用武火煮沸后，转用文火炖 1 小时即成，食莲子、百合、猪肉，喝汤。

功效：清心除烦，宁心安神。

适宜人群：心烦，失眠多梦，长期腹泻、稀便，男性遗精，腰膝酸软，女性白带夹血丝者，以及咳嗽、痰中带血、体虚心烦不安者。

Diet therapy: Stewed Pork with Lotus Seeds and Lily

Ingredients: Lotus seeds 50 g, lily 50 g, pork 200g, appropriate amount of salt, green onion and ginger.

Methods: Chop the pork into small pieces, then add lotus seeds, lily and water with salt, green onion, and ginger. Bring to a boil and simmer for another one hour.

Actions: Clearing the heart and relieving vexation, calming the mind.

Indicated population: Those with vexation, insomnia with profuse dreaming, chronic diarrhea, loose stool, and cough with blood-tinged phlegm, and restlessness. Male with spermatorrhea and soreness and weakness of the lower back and knees; and female with blood-tinged leukorrhea.

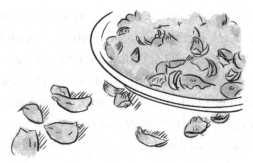

大暑 Greater Heat (Dashu)

大暑为每年公历 7 月 23 日前后，太阳黄经为 120°。大暑是一年中最热的节气，正值中伏前后，我国长江流域的许多地方常出现 40℃的高温。大暑雨水多，应注意防汛防涝。

Each year around July 23rd when the sun reaches celestial longitude of 120°, the solar term of *Greater Heat* (Dashu) arrives. It marks the hottest days of the year, exactly in the second ten-day period of the dog days. The temperature might reach 40 ℃ in most of the Yangtze River region. Since there is increased rainfall in this solar term, prevention of flood and waterlog should be emphasized.

【大暑防中暑是关键】
Heatstroke prevention being essential

❶ 中暑的症状

中暑分先兆中暑、轻度中暑和重度中暑。先兆中暑表现为大量出汗、口渴、四肢无力、恶心等，体温正常或略高，一般不超过37.5℃；轻度中暑表现为面色潮红、头痛、胸闷、多汗、口渴、心慌乏力等，体温升高到38℃以上，血压下降、脉搏加快等；重度中暑除上述症状外，可能还会出现昏倒或痉挛，或皮肤干燥无汗，体温在40℃以上。

❶ Symptoms of heatstroke

Heatstroke can be divided into aura of heatstroke, mild heatstroke and severe heatstroke. Aura of heatstroke involves symptoms of profuse sweating, thirst, weak limbs, nausea, and normal or slightly high temperature that rarely exceeds 37.5 ℃. In addition to profuse sweating and thirst, mild heatstroke also manifests as flushed cheeks, headache, chest tightness, palpitations, lack of strength, high temperature that reaches above 38 ℃, dropped blood pressure, and increased pulse. Severe heatstroke includes more than the above symptoms, such as coma or spasm, or dry skin, and temperature over 40 ℃.

❷ 中暑的高发人群

中暑的高发人群主要包括在高温下作业、晒又无法及时补充水分的人群，体质较差的老年人、儿童，以及本身患有糖尿病、心脑血管疾病、代谢性疾病等基础疾病的患者。还有一些长期在低温空调室内，突然进入室外高温环境的人群。

❷High risk population

It mainly includes those who work in high temperature, unable to replenish water in time yet exposed to the blazing sun for quite a long time, and those with poor constitution, such as the elderly, children, and patients with other basic diseases like diabetes, cardiovascular and cerebrovascular diseases and metabolic diseases. Those who stay in a room of low temperature with air conditioner on for a long time are also liable to heatstroke when suddenly going out where the temperature is very high.

❸ 中暑的处置

迅速撤离引起中暑的高温环境，选择阴凉通风的地方休息。多饮用一些含盐分的清凉饮料，也可在额部、颞部涂抹清凉油、风油精等，或服用人丹、十滴水、藿香正气水等中药。如果出现血压降低、虚脱时应立即平卧，及时送到医院治疗。

❸Management

Move the person from high-temperature environment that causes heatstroke to an air-conditioned and shady environment. Provide them with drinks that contain salt. Cooling balm or medicated oil can be applied on the forehead and temples. Chinese medicines fo heatstroke can be used, such as Rendan Pills, Shidishui Oral Liquid, Agastache Qi-Correcting Oral Liquid, etc. Lay the person down when there is blood pressure drop and prostration, and transport him or her to the hospital as soon as possible.

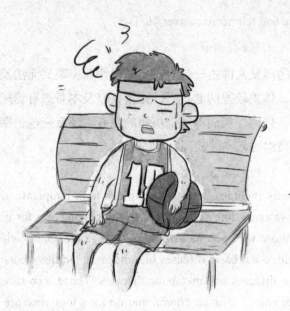

❹ 中暑预防

做好外出前准备工作

①夏季外出时要备好防晒用具和做好防护工作。老年人、孕妇、慢性疾病患者，特别是有心血管疾病者尽可能减少外出活动。②衣服尽量选用棉、麻、丝类的织物，应少穿化纤类服装。③准备充足的水、饮料和防暑降温药品，如人丹、十滴水、风油精等，以备应急之用。

❹ Prevention of summer-heat stroke

Preparations before going out

①Sun protection should be emphasized before going out in summer. The elderly, pregnant women, patients with chronic diseases, especially cardiovascular diseases, should reduce their outdoor activities as much as possible. ②Choose clothes made of cotton, linen and silk fabrics rather than chemical fibers. ③Prepare enough water, drinks and medicines that can reduce heat and prevent heatstroke, such as Rendan Pills, Shidishui Oral Liquid, and medicated oil, etc.

保证充足的水分

①高温作业人员应及时补充水分，多饮清凉盐开水、绿豆汤、

酸梅汤等，弥补人体因出汗而失去的盐分。

Adequate water intake

①Those who work in high temperature should replenish water in time, and drink more cool salt water, Mung Bean Soup, Sour Plum Drink, etc. to make up for the loss of salt due to sweating.

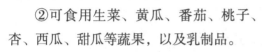

②可食用生菜、黄瓜、番茄、桃子、杏、西瓜、甜瓜等蔬果，以及乳制品。

②Vegetables and fruits such as lettuce, cucumber, tomato, peach, apricot, watermelon, muskmelon etc., and diary products can be taken.

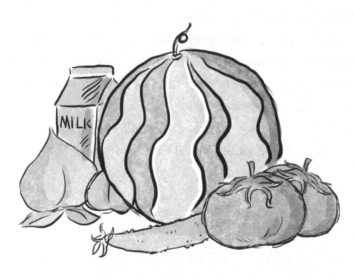

合理安排工作

大暑时节，要合理安排作息时间，做到早出工、晚收工，适当延长中午休息时间。

Appropriate work schedule

It is important to arrange work schedule appropriately in Greater

Heat. You should go to work early and return late to avoid the heat, and remember to prolong the lunch break properly.

【大暑食疗方：荷叶薄荷粥】

材料：鲜荷叶 1 张，薄荷 30g，粳米 100g，冰糖适量。

做法：将鲜荷叶洗净、切碎，薄荷洗净，两物加适量清水用中火煮后取汁，倒入粳米煮粥，然后加冰糖，即可食用。

功效：清热消暑。

适宜人群：心烦口渴、食欲不佳、食少腹胀者。

Diet therapy: Porridge of Lotus Leaves and Mint

Ingredients: A piece of fresh lotus leaf, mint 30g, japonica rice 100g, appropriate amount of rock sugar.

Methods: Wash and cut up the lotus leaf, and boil it with rinsed mint and appropriate amount of water with medium heat. Combine the decocted juice with japonica rice and add rock sugar before eating.

Actions: Clearing summer-heat.

Indicated population: Those with vexation and thirst, poor appetite, little intake of food and abdominal distension.

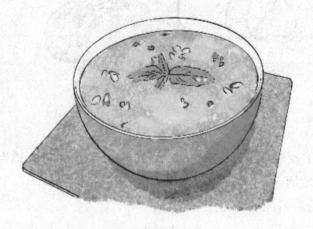

秋季 AUTUMN

秋三月，起于立秋，止于立冬前。秋季分为立秋、处暑、白露、秋分、寒露、霜降六个节气。

秋季是夏冬两季的过渡时期，气温由热向寒转变，空气湿度降低，昼夜温差增大，北方受冷空气侵入，天气凉爽，南方常有绵绵秋雨出现。

秋季天气转凉，衣被添加进度应缓，可有意识地让身体"冻一冻"，尤其是老年人。

There are three months in autumn, starting with *Beginning of Autumn* (Liqiu) and ending before *Beginning of Winter* (Lidong), divided into six solar terms of Beginning of Autumn, *End of Heat* (Chushu), *White Dew* (Bailu), *Autumn Equinox* (Qiufen), *Cold Dew* (Hanlu) and *First Frost* (Shuangjiang).

Autumn is the transitional period between summer and winter. In Autumn, the temperature gradually drops, the air humidity gradually decreases and diurnal temperature range gradually increases. In northern areas, the weather is cool due to the invasion of cold air and in southern areas, there is often continuous rain.

As the weather turns cooler in autumn, there is no need to add clothes and quilts too quickly, so the body can gradually adapt to the cold air, especially for the elderly.

宜：润肺和"酸味"的食物，如山药、莲藕、杏仁及山楂、柚子、石榴等。

Recommended: lung-moistening foods, such as yam, lotus root, almonds, etc.; foods which are sour in flavor, such as Chinese hawthorn fruit, pomelo, pomegranate, etc.

不宜：葱、姜、蒜、韭菜、芥末等辛味食物。

Not recommended: foods which are pungent in flavor, such as green onion, ginger, garlic, Chinese chives and mustard, etc.

饮食

【宜润肺忌寒凉】

要以防秋燥、滋阴润肺为基本原则，宜食润肺的食物，如蜂蜜、梨、百合、莲子、银耳、木耳等食物。少食寒凉性水果，如西瓜、山竹等。同时，要多喝温水，每天应适时饮水，饮水量可达到2500mL。

Moistening the lung and avoiding cold

With "preventing autumn dryness, nourishing yin and moistening the lung" as the basic principle, it is recommended to eat lung-moistening foods, such as honey, pear, lily, lotus seeds, snow fungus, wood ear, etc. The intake of fruits which are cold in property should be decreased, such as watermelon, mangosteen, etc. What's more, it's recommended to drink more warm water for 2500 mL every day at appropriate time.

【 忌随意"贴秋膘" 】

一到秋季，民间流行"贴秋膘"，以储备热量，应对冬季的寒冷。但秋天不宜随意进补，以免加重脾胃负担，引起消化功能紊乱，尤其是脾胃功能较弱的老年人和儿童要注意不可随意"贴秋膘"。

Be careful of "putting on weight in autumn"

Once autumn arrives, it is popular to "put on weight in autumn" in order to reserve heat to cope with the cold winter. However, it is not advisable to tonify at will in autumn, as it will impose burden on the spleen and stomach and lead to digestive disorders, especially for the elderly and children with weak spleen and stomach functions.

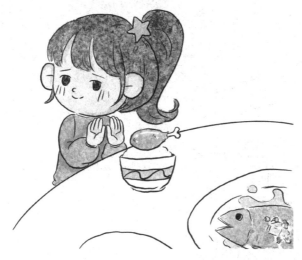

睡眠

经过漫长、炎热的夏季，人体易出现体液平衡失调、肠胃功能减弱、心血管系统负担加重等，而使身体处于过度消耗的状态。进入秋季，人体则进入了一个周期性的休整阶段，为更好地适应季节变化，睡眠应注意以下几点。

The past long hot summer increases the risk of imbalance of body fluids, weakened gastrointestinal function, increased burden on the cardiovascular system, etc., and the body is in a state of overconsumption. As autumn arrives, the human body enters a cyclical resting stage in order to adapt to seasonal changes better. As for sleep, people should pay attention to the following tips.

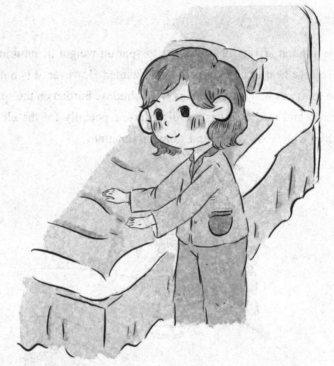

【晚上 11 点前睡】

秋季万物萧条，人的起居在此时应随气候进行相应的调整。尤其入夜之后，气温下降快，应早睡早起，尽量在晚上 11 时前睡觉，早晨早起床。

In autumn, everything is depressed, and the time to get up and go to bed should be adjusted according to the climate. Especially at night when the temperature drops quickly, it's better to go to bed before 11 pm and get up early.

【选对被褥】

秋季天气逐渐变凉，盖被不需要太厚，建议选择质地轻薄易保暖兼有吸湿吸汗之功效的羽绒被。

Choosing the right bedding

The temperature gradually drops in autumn, but the quilt does not need to be too thick, and it is recommended to choose the duvet which is light and easy to keep warm and absorb moisture and sweat.

【忌开窗正对风口睡眠】

秋夜天凉，开窗正对风口睡觉易使人感到头昏脑涨，甚至引起偏头痛等。尽量不要开窗睡觉，睡前开窗通风即可。

秋季 AUTUMN

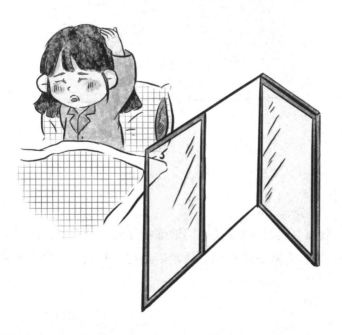

79

Avoiding sleeping in front of the opening window

In autumn, it's cool at night, so sleeping with the window open can easily lead to dizziness and even migraines. It's better not to sleep with the window open, and just open the window before going to bed to ventilate.

【脚部保暖】

脚部被称为人体的第二心脏，在脚部有众多的穴位及经脉，秋季夜晚气温低，睡觉时要注意脚部保暖，以确保血液循环，尤其是心脏血液的流动顺畅。

Keeping feet warm

Feet are conceived as the body's second heart as there are numerous acupoints and meridians. In autumn, it's cold at night, so keep feet warm when sleeping to ensure smooth blood circulation, especially the blood circulation of heart.

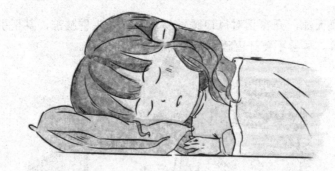

活动

"秋高气爽"，秋季是人们锻炼身体的黄金季节，每天活动 30 分钟左右，有益身体健康。活动时最好选择透气、散湿性较好的衣服，活动前 2 小时可先喝水 300 ～ 500mL。具体推荐以下几项活动。

With the clear sky and fresh air, autumn is suitable for people to exercise. It's beneficial for health to exercise about 30 minutes every day, wearing clothes with good breathability and drinking 300-500 mL of water 2 hours before the exercises. The following activities are recommended.

【 爬山 】

爬山能增加肺通气量和肺活量，增强血液循环。建议每周爬山 1 次，每次 30 ～ 60 分钟，每爬 20 分钟，最好休息几分钟。此外，气温较低时，可以戴一个护膝，但切忌太紧；爬山后注意保暖，可以通过热敷、泡脚等方式改善关节酸痛。禁忌人群：①患有运动障碍慢性疾病者，如关节病等；②患有呼吸系统慢性疾病者，如严重的肺心病、慢性气管炎等；③患有循环系统慢性疾病者，如高血压、冠心病、慢性冠状动脉供血不足等；④患有其他疾病者，如慢性肾炎、血液病、糖尿病伴有并发症、痛风、红斑狼疮等。

Climbing mountains

Lung ventilation and capacity could be increased and blood circulation could be improved through climbing mountains. It is recommended to climb once a week, 30-60 minutes each time. It is suggested to take a break every 20 minutes. In addition, when the temperature is low, it is better to wear a knee brace which should not be too tight. Remember to keep warm afterwards. Besides, joint pain can be relieved through hot compresses, foot soaks and other ways.

Contraindicated population:

①people with chronic diseases of movement disorders, such as joint diseases.

②people with chronic diseases of the respiratory system, such as severe pulmonary heart disease, chronic bronchitis, etc..

③people with chronic diseases of the circulatory system, such as hypertension, coronary heart disease, chronic coronary insufficiency, etc..

④people with other diseases, such as chronic nephritis, blood diseases, diabetes with comorbidities, gout, lupus erythematosus, etc.

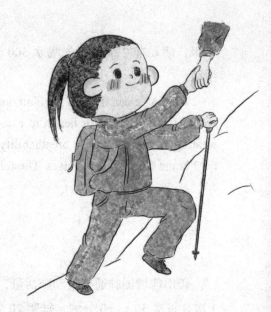

【长跑】

长跑[1]能增强血液循环，改善心功能、脑的血液供应和脑细胞的氧供应，还能有效地刺激代谢，增加能量消耗。建议每周坚持2次长跑，每次跑5km以上。禁忌人群：①有潜藏疾病者，主要是心脑血管疾病；②平时无体育锻炼者，如果运动量大大超出平时负荷，产生运动过度紧张，可能会造成猝死或者其他运动伤害；③轻度活动就有胸闷、头痛、头晕等不适症状者；④老年高血压和糖尿病患者。

Long-distance running

Long-distance running[1] can stimulate blood circulation, improve heart function, blood and oxygen supply to the brain, and also effectively stimulate metabolism and increase energy consumption. It is recommended to insist on long-distance running twice a week for more than 5 km each time.

Contraindicated population

①people with latent diseases, such as cardiovascular and cerebrovascular diseases.

②people without physical exercise. Exercise-induced overstrain would be brought out due to over-exercise, which may lead to sudden death or other sports injuries.

③people with chest tightness, headache, dizziness and other discomfort symptoms after mild activity.

④elderly patients with hypertension and diabetes.

[1] 长跑：指路程为 5km 及以上的长距离跑步。

[1] Long-distance running: running with a distance of 5 km or more.

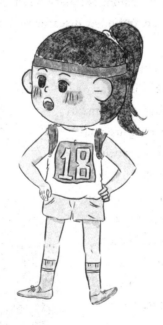

【骑行】

骑行能预防大脑老化，提高神经系统的敏捷性，还能提高心肺功能，锻炼下肢肌力，增强全身耐力。每周坚持 2 ～ 3 次骑行，每次 3 ～ 5km。需要注意的：①高血压、冠心病、疝气、癫痫、脑震荡后遗症等疾病患者不宜骑行；②男性不适合将骑行当做长期锻炼的项目，这是因为自行车车座窄小，若长时间骑行，男性睾丸、前列腺等器官会因受到长期挤压而出现缺血、水肿、发炎等症状；③正处于生长发育阶段的青少年也不适宜骑行，若选用车把较低的自行车长时间骑行，可能会影响脊柱的弯曲度，影响形体发育。

Cycling

Cycling can prevent brain aging, improve the agility of the nervous system, and also improve cardiorespiratory function, exercise muscle strength of lower limbs, and enhance endurance. It is recommended to ride 2 to 3 times a week, 3 to 5 km each time.

The following things should be noted

①Patients with hypertension, coronary heart disease, hernia, epilepsy, concussion sequelae and other diseases patients are not recommended to cycle.

②Men are not suitable for cycling as a long-term exercise, because ischemia, edema, inflammation and other symptoms of testicles, prostate and other organs would be induced after a long-time extrusion due to the long-time cycling.

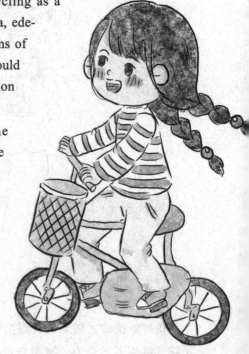

③Adolescents who are in the growth and development stage are also not suitable for cycling, because long-time cycling with low-handle-bar bike may affect the curvature of the spine and finally affect the physical development.

穴位养生

进入秋季，空气逐渐干燥，此时最容易造成肺的损伤，因此，秋季宜养肺润肺。

As autumn comes, lung is easy to be hurt due to the dry air at this time. Therefore, it is better to nourish and moisten the lung in autumn.

迎香穴

【位置】位于鼻翼旁约 0.2cm 的鼻唇沟中。

【功效】养肺润肺。

【方法】将两手拇指外侧相互摩擦，有热感后，用拇指外侧沿鼻梁、鼻翼两侧上下按摩约 60 次后再按摩鼻翼两侧的迎香穴 20 次，每天早晚各做 1 ～ 2 组。

Yingxiang (LI 20)

Location: In the nasolabial fold, about 0.2 cm next to the nose wing.

Actions: Nourishing and moistening the lung.

Methods: Rub the lateral thumbs against each other, and when the skin feels warm, massage along both sides of the bridge and the nose wing up and down about 60 times with the lateral thumbs and then massage Yingxiang (LI 20) 20 times a day, 1 to 2 groups in each morning and evening.

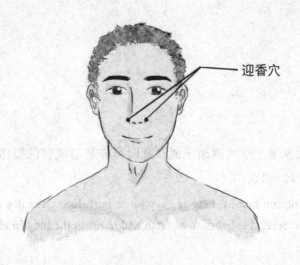

迎香穴

肺俞穴

【位置】位于背后第三胸椎棘突下，左右旁约两指宽处。

【功效】可舒畅胸中之气，健肺养肺，且可疏通脊背经脉，预防感冒。

【方法】每晚临睡前端坐在椅子上，两膝自然分开，双手放在大腿上，头正目闭，全身放松。吸气于胸中，两手握成空心拳，轻叩肺俞穴数十下，同时用手掌在背部两侧由下至上轻拍，持续约10分钟。也可艾炷灸5～7壮，艾条灸10～20分钟，局部有温热感为度。

Feishu (BL 13)

Location: Two fingers width lateral to the spinous process of the 3rd thoracic vertebra.

Actions: Soothing the qi in the chest, invigorating and nourishing the lung, and also freeing the meridians on the back to prevent cold.

Methods: Every night before going to bed, sit on a chair with knees naturally apart, hands on your thighs, head straight, eyes closed, and the whole body relaxed. Inhale and tap on Feishu (BL 13) gently for dozens of times with hollow fists, while patting with the palms on both sides of the back from bottom to top for about 10 minutes. Moxibustion of 5 to 7 cones, or moxibustion with moxa sticks for 10 to 20 minutes is recommended until there is local warmth.

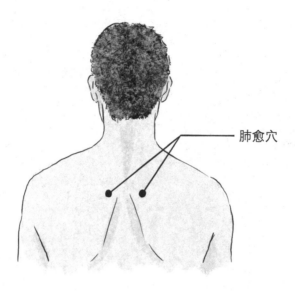

肺愈穴

列缺穴

【位置】双手虎口平直交叉，一手食指按在另一手桡骨茎突上，指尖下凹陷处即为列缺穴。

【功效】调理肺气，常用于治疗咳嗽、气喘、慢性阻塞性肺疾病等。

【方法】可将艾绒捏成麦粒状，放置于列缺穴上点燃，待皮肤有温热感时取下，再放置下一粒，每次 5 ～ 7 粒，每周 1 ～ 2 次。

Lieque (LU 7)

Location: Interlock your thumb and index finger of one hand with those of the other and press the index finger of one hand on the styloid process of the radius. The depression under the fingertip is Lieque.

Actions: Regulating the lung qi, which is suitable for cough, asthma, chronic obstructive pulmonary disease, etc.

Methods: Knead the moxa into cones like wheat seeds, place it on Lieque and ignite it, and replace it with another one when the skin feels warm, 5-7 grains each time, once or twice a week.

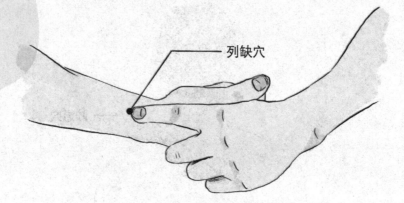

列缺穴

立秋 Beginning of Autumn (Liqiu)

立秋一般在每年公历 8 月 8 日前后，太阳黄经为 135°。立秋预示着炎热的夏季即将过去，秋季即将来临。立秋后，气温逐渐下降。

In the Gregorian calendar, *Beginning of Autumn* (Liqiu) usually begins around August 8 when the sun reaches the celestial longitude of 135°, which indicates that the hot summer is coming to an end and autumn is approaching. After *Beginning of Autumn*, the temperature gradually drops.

【立秋以养肺为主】Mainly nourishing the lung

❶ 最佳养肺时间：上午 7 ~ 9 时

此时是肺功能最强之时，此时进行慢跑等运动，能强健肺功能，但患有高血压、心脏疾病、气喘等人群，应适当减少运动量。

❶The best lung-nourishing time: 7-9 am.

From 7 to 9 am, the function of lung is the strongest. At this time, jogging and other sports can strengthen its function, but people with hypertension, heart disease, asthma and other diseases should appropriately exercise less.

❷ 最简单养肺法：用一杯热水

将热水倒入茶杯中，用鼻子对准茶杯吸入水蒸汽，每次约 10 分钟，可早晚各 1 次，可有润肺之效。

❷The simplest lung-nourishing method: a cup of hot water.

Pour hot water into the tea cup, inhale water vapor for about 10 minutes each time, twice a day in the morning and evening, which can moisten the lung.

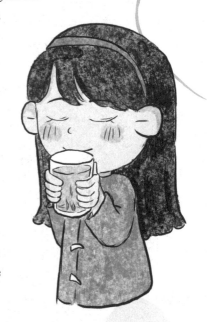

❸ 最有效养肺法：主动咳嗽

立秋后，每日早晚可选择面对空气清新处，深呼吸后主动咳嗽，以清除呼吸道及肺部吸入的粉尘、有害气体、金属微粒及工业废气中的毒性物质等，减少对肺部的损害。

❸The most effective lung-nourishing method: cough by yourself.

After *Beginning of Autumn*, take a deep breath of the fresh air every morning and evening, and then cough by yourself to remove the dust, harmful gases, metal particles and toxic substances of industrial waste gas from the respiratory tract and lungs, so as to reduce the damage to the lung.

❹ 最便捷的养肺法：笑口常开

大笑能使肺扩张，大笑的同时还会不自觉地进行深呼吸，使呼吸更通畅。

❹The most convenient lung-nourishing method: smile.

Laughter can expand the lung. While laughing, we would take a deep breath and have better breathing.

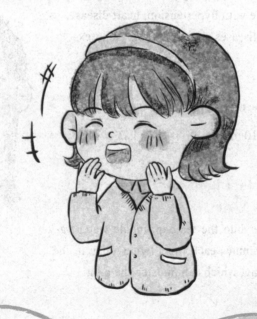

【立秋养生食疗方：百合杏仁粥】

材料：百合 10g，杏仁 6g，粳米 100g，白糖少许。

做法：先将粳米以武火煮沸，然后在半熟的粳米锅内加入百合、杏仁、白糖，以文火煮沸即成。

功效：滋阴润肺，清心安神。

适宜人群：咳喘、便秘、失眠心烦、多梦者。

Health-nurturing recipe: Lily Almond Porridge

Ingredients: Lily 10 g, almond 6 g, japonica rice 100g, a little white sugar.

Methods: Boil the japonica rice with strong fire, then add lily, almond and white sugar into the half-cooked japonica rice, and finally boil the porridge with mild fire.

Actions: Nourishing yin and moistening the lung; clearing the heart and tranquilizing mind.

Indicated population: Those with cough, panting, constipation, insomnia, vexation and dreamfulness.

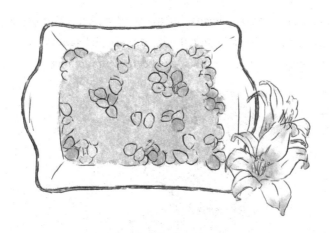

处暑 End of Heat (Chushu)

处暑一般在每年公历 8 月 23 日前后，太阳黄经为 150°，处暑即为 "出暑"，意味着即将进入气象意义的秋天，处暑后，我国黄河以北气温逐渐下降。

In the Gregorian calendar, *End of Heat* (Chushu) usually begins around August 23 when the sun reaches the celestial longitude of 150°, which means "end of heat" and indicates that meteorological autumn is coming. After End of Heat, the temperature in the north of the Yellow River gradually drops.

【处暑防燥是关键】

❶ 皮肤干燥，浑身瘙痒

处暑后皮脂腺、汗腺分泌减少，加上空气干燥，皮肤易失去水分，而出现脱皮、瘙痒等症状。

Preventing dryness as the key

❶ Dry skin, and itching

After *End of Heat*, because of the reduced secretion of sebaceous glands and sweat glands, coupled with dry air, the skin is easy to dehydrate, and there are symptoms such as peeling and itching.

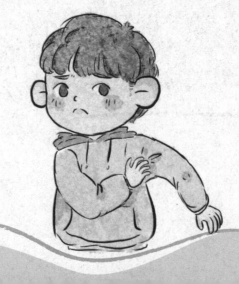

预防：多饮水，多食用苹果、柚子、橘子等水果，室内可使用加湿器，将湿度调节到 40% ～ 60%。除特殊情况外，尽量避免每天洗澡，可隔天洗一次，洗澡时水温控制在 34 ～ 36℃，时间不宜超过 5 分钟。

Prevention: Drink more water, eat more fruits such as apples, pomelo and oranges, and use humidifiers indoors to adjust the humidity to 40% to 60%. Except for special cases, try to take a bath every other day instead of bathing daily, control the water temperature at 34℃ to 36℃ and limit the shower time within 5 minutes.

❷ 上火、便秘、眼睛干涩、流鼻血

处暑后身体易缺水，鼻腔黏膜干燥，易引起上火、便秘、眼睛干涩、流鼻血等症状。

预防：除清淡饮食外，每天应喝水 2500mL，另外可使用防裂唇膏滋润鼻腔，并在医生指导下使用眼药膏来滋润眼睛。

❷ Excessive internal heat, constipation, dry eyes, nosebleeds

After *End of Heat*, lack of water may induce excessive internal heat, constipation, dry eyes, dry nasal mucosa and even nosebleed and other symptoms.

Prevention: In addition to a light diet, drink 2500 mL water a day, use lip balm to moisten the nasal cavity, and use eye ointment to moisten the eyes under the guidance of doctors.

❸ 口角干裂

处暑后气候干燥，口角周围皮肤黏膜易干裂，病菌乘虚而入造成感染，从而引发口角炎。

秋季 AUTUMN

93

❸ Dry and cracked labial angles

After *End of Heat*, dryness is easy to induce dry and cracked skin around the mouth and then it may lead to angular stomatitis because of bacterial infection.

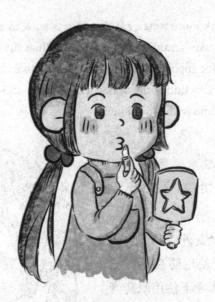

预防： 多食用富含 B 族维生素的食物，如瘦肉、禽蛋、牛奶、豆制品、胡萝卜、新鲜绿叶蔬菜等。口角干裂时，可使用润唇膏滋润嘴唇，不要舔唇，以免加重口角干裂，进一步诱发口角炎。

Prevention: Eat more food rich in B vitamins, such as lean meat, eggs, milk, bean products, carrots, fresh green leafy vegetables, etc. Lip balms can be used to moisten the dry and cracked lips. Do not lick the lips, so as not to aggravate the symptom and further induce angular stomatitis.

【处暑养生食疗方：沙参粥】

材料： 沙参 15～30g，粳米 50g，冰糖适量。

做法： 先将沙参捣碎，加水煎取药汁后去渣，然后将药汁与粳米同入砂锅，再加水适量，以文火煮粥，待粥煮沸时，加入冰糖稍煮片刻即可。

功效：养阴清肺，益胃生津。

适宜人群：干咳、声音嘶哑、咽干舌燥者。

Health-nurturing recipe: Adenophora Porridge

Ingredients: Adenophora root (Shashen) 15-30g, japonica rice 50g, and appropriate amount of rock sugar.

Methods: Mash the adenophora root, add water to decoct and remove the dregs, then put the decoction into the casserole with japonica rice, cook the porridge with mild fire after adding appropriate amount of water again, and when the porridge boils, add rock sugar and cook for a moment.

Actions: Nourishing yin and clearing the lung; boosting the stomach and engendering liquid.

Indicated population: Those with dry cough, hoarse voice and dry throat.

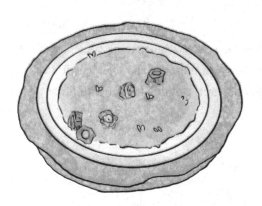

白露 White Dew (Bailu)

　　白露一般在每年公历 9 月 8 日前后，太阳黄经为 165°。白露后秋意渐浓，天气转凉，昼夜温差可达 10℃。

　　In the Gregorian calendar, *White Dew* (Bailu) usually begins around September 8th when the sun reaches the celestial longitude of 165°. After *White Dew*, the atmosphere of autumn is getting stronger, with the cooler weather. The temperature differences between day and night can reach up to 10℃

【白露养生做好"三防"】
"Three preventions" for health nurturing

❶ 防凉：白露身不露

　　白露后，天气转凉，早晚温差较大，如果衣着过于单薄或者裸露四肢，极易诱发感冒或导致旧疾复发。

❶Prevention of cold: Keeping dressing warm

After *White Dew*, the weather turns cooler with the large temperature difference between morning and evening. It's easy to induce colds or relapses without warm clothing thin or with limbs uncovered.

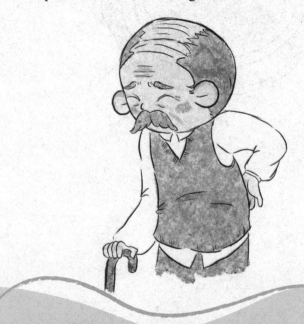

❷ 防病：心脑血管疾病

白露早晚温差进一步加大，心脑血管疾病患者应在医生指导下根据病情调整用药，并注意休息，做好保暖工作，避免感冒诱发急性心脑血管疾病。抵抗力不佳的中老年人也要注意防护，以免因早晚低温使外周血管收缩、血压升高而诱发心脑血管疾病。

❷Prevention of disease: cardiovascular and cerebro-vascular diseases

With the vast temperature difference between morning and evening further increases, patients with cardiovascular and cerebrovascular diseases should adjust their medication according to their conditions under the guidance of doctors and pay attention to rest and keep warm to avoid acute cardiovascular and cerebrovascular diseases induced by colds. Middle-aged and elderly people with poor immunity should also pay attention to protection, so as not to contract such diseases due to peripheral vasoconstriction and elevated blood pressure caused by low temperatures in the morning and evening.

❸ 防悲：谨防悲秋来袭

白露后，花草树木开始凋谢，人们易触景伤情，此时应多与他人沟通交流，保持愉快舒畅的心情。

❸Prevention of sadness: Guarding against sadness

After *White Dew*, as flowers and trees begin to wither, people are easy to be sad due to such scene. At this time, it's better to talk to others to maintain a happy and relaxed mood.

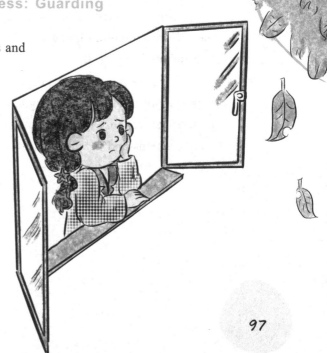

【白露养生食疗方：黄芪三七鸡】

材料：黄芪 60g，三七 10g，仔母鸡 1 只，料酒 10g，盐适量。

做法：把黄芪洗净切片，放入砂锅，再将干净的仔母鸡加进砂锅，加水 1500mL，加料酒，武火煮沸，撇去浮沫，加盐少许，文火炖至鸡肉烂熟后再去掉黄芪、三七等渣。

功效：补气健脾，活血化瘀。

适宜人群：浑身无力、食少稀便、水肿、咳嗽、哮喘、骨折后期恢复者。

Health-nurturing recipe: Stewed Chicken with Astragalus and Notoginseng

Ingredients: Astragalus (Huangqi) 60g, notoginseng (Sanqi) 10g, one poussin hen, cooking wine 10 g, and appropriate amount of salt.

Methods: Put the washed and sliced astragalus and clean poussin hen into the casserole, add 1500 mL of water, and cooking wine, bring to a boil with strong fire, and then skim the foam, add a pinch of salt. Remove astragalus, notoginseng and other dregs after the chicken is well cooked with mild fire.

Actions: Tonifying qi and strengthening the spleen; promoting blood circulation and resolving stasis.

Indicated population: People with symptoms of lack of strength, poor appetite, loose stool, edema, cough, asthma and people who are recovering from fracture.

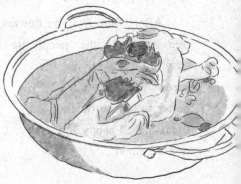

秋分 Autumn Equinox (Qiufen)

秋分为每年公历 9 月 23 日前后，太阳黄经为 180°。秋分当日，北半球昼夜几乎相等，秋分后，太阳直射位置继续由赤道向南半球推移，昼短夜长的趋势愈发明显。

In the Gregorian calendar, *Autumn Equinox* (Qiufen) usually begins around September 23rd when the sun reaches the celestial longitude of 180°. On Autumnal Equinox, the day and night in the northern hemisphere are almost equal. However, after that, the position of direct sunlight continues to move from the equator to the southern hemisphere, and the days are shorter and nights are longer.

【秋分保护好六个部位】Protecting six body parts

❶ 头部

寒冷空气若入侵头部，易引起感冒、鼻炎、头痛、牙痛、三叉神经痛等。

预防：在气温突降而需要外出时，可戴上帽子，为头部保暖。每天清晨可梳头百余次，使头皮微热，有利于头部气血通畅。秋分时，晚上最好不要洗头。

❶ Head

If cold air invades the head, it is easy to cause cold, rhinitis, headache, toothache, trigeminal neuralgia, etc.

Prevention: If you need to go out when the temperature drops suddenly, you can wear a hat to keep your head warm. You can comb your hair more than 100 times every morning to make the scalp slightly hot, which is

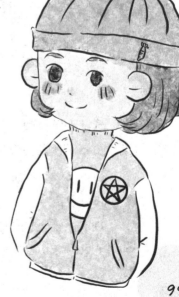

conducive to the smooth flow of qi and blood in the head. However, on the *Autumnal Equinox*, it's better not to wash your hair at night.

❷ 口鼻

口鼻是空气进出的通道，寒气进入肺部，易出现恶心、呕吐、咳嗽、吐痰、鼻塞、打喷嚏等。

预防：空气质量不好时，出行建议戴口罩加强防护，平时注意清理呼吸道，避免异物或粉尘刺激口鼻。

❷Mouth and nose

Mouth and nose are the passages of air. If cold air enters the lungs, it is easy to cause nausea, vomiting, cough, expectoration, nasal congestion, sneezing, etc.

Prevention: If there is poor air quality, it is recommended to wear masks and pay attention to cleaning the respiratory tract to avoid foreign matters or dust that could stimulate the mouth and nose.

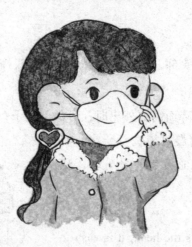

❸ 颈部

颈部上承头颅，下接躯干，是人体的要塞。颈部受凉，易使大脑供血不足诱发头晕等症状。

预防：穿立领装，外出戴围巾。

❸Neck

The neck, the bridge of the head and the trunk, is the fortress of the human body. Cold invasion of the neck can easily lead to dizziness and other symptoms due to insufficient blood supply to the brain.

Prevention: Wear clothing with standing collar and scarf when going out.

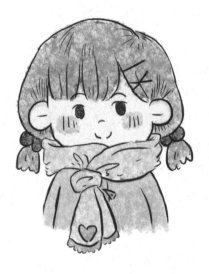

❹ 腰部

腰部受寒，易引发疼痛，导致全身乏力。

预防：双手搓腰，两手对搓发热后，按摩腰部早晚各 1 次，每次 50 ～ 100 遍。

❹Waist

Cold invasion of the waist can easily trigger pain, resulting in general weakness.

Prevention: Rub the waist with both warm hands every morning and evening, 50 to 100 times each time.

❺ 背部

背部受寒，时间一长可引起颈椎病、肩周炎、腰椎间盘突出、腰肌劳损及慢性腰腿痛等。

预防：注意背部的防寒和保暖。

❺Back

Cold on the back for a long time can cause cervical spondylosis, scapulohumeral periarthritis, lumbar herniated disk, lumbar muscle strain, chronic pain in the low back and legs, etc.

Prevention: Pay attention to keeping the back warm.

【秋分养生食疗方：天门冬粥】

材料：天冬 20g，粳米 100g，冰糖适量。

做法：将天冬捣碎，放入砂锅内，加水煎取浓汁，去渣；将粳米洗净，放入砂锅内，加适量水，大火煮沸，改为小火煮约 30 分钟成粥，加入冰糖调味即成。

功效：滋补润肺，养肺生津。

适宜人群：干咳痰少、咽喉痛、声音嘶哑、眩晕、耳鸣、腰膝酸软及便秘者。

Health-nurturing recipe: Asparagus Porridge

Ingredients: Asparagus (Tianmendong) 20g, japonica rice 100g, and appropriate amount of rock sugar.

Methods: Mash asparagus, put it into a casserole, add water to decoct, and get the juice without dregs; Wash the japonica rice, put it into a casserole, add appropriate amount of water, bring to a boil over strong fire, and simmer for about 30 minutes, then add rock sugar.

Actions: Nourishing and moistening the lung to engender liquid.

Indicated population: Those manifesting as dry cough with little phlegm, sore throat, hoarseness, dizziness, tinnitus, soreness and weakness of the waist and knees, and constipation.

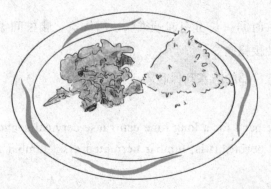

寒露 Cold Dew (Hanlu)

寒露一般为每年公历 10 月 9 日前后，太阳黄经为 195°。寒露后，天气从凉爽向寒冷过渡，气温更低了。

In the Gregorian calendar, *Cold Dew* (Hanlu) usually begins around October 9th when the sun reaches the celestial longitude of 195°. After *Cold Dew*, the weather changes from cool to cold, as the temperatures drop further.

【寒露养生驱寒为主】
Mainly dispelling cold for health nurturing

❶ 足部保暖

寒露过后，气温逐渐降低，此时要注意足部保暖，选用质地舒适、保暖效果好的鞋袜。同时，可以每天晚上睡觉前采用热水泡脚，泡脚能促进足部的血管扩张、血流加快，缓解疲劳。建议泡脚时长 40 分钟，水温控制在 40℃左右，可加入生姜、陈皮等。

❶ Keeping feet warm

After *Cold Dew*, as the temperature gradually drops, attention should be paid to feet warmth by choosing shoes and socks with comfortable texture and good thermal effect. Moreover, it is recommended to soak your feet in water at about 40℃ every night before going to bed for 40 minutes to promote the vasodilation of feet, accelerate blood flow and relieve fatigue. Ginger, tangerine peel and others can be added into water.

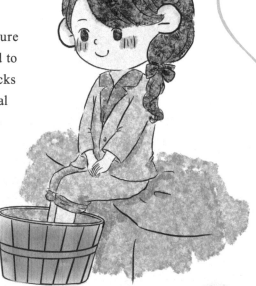

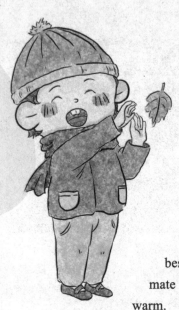

❷ 适时添衣

寒露后，老年人、儿童和体质较弱者应逐渐增添衣服，最好厚薄搭配，以保暖为主。

❷Adding clothes in time

After Cold Dew, the elderly, children and people with weak constitution should gradually add clothes. It is best to choose clothes according to the climate and priority should be given to keeping warm.

❸ 轻松活动

寒露时进行轻松的活动有利于改善血液循环，对消化吸收能力也有帮助，如慢跑、瑜伽等。

❸Relaxing exercise

During Cold Dew, relaxing activities can improve blood circulation, digestion and absorption capacity, such as jogging or doing yoga.

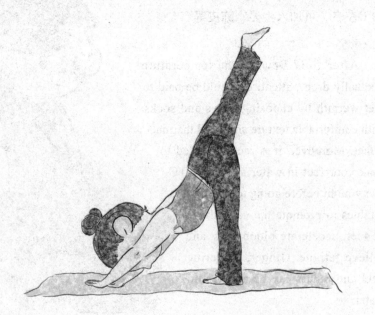

【 寒露养生食疗方：川贝炖雪梨 】

材料：雪梨 800g，川贝 10g，冰糖 10g。

做法：将雪梨去皮去核后与川贝同放入碗内，加入冰糖炖 1 小时左右即可。

功效：润肺止咳。

适宜人群：干咳无痰、久咳者。

Health-nurturing recipe: Stewed Snow Pear with Sichuan Scallop

Ingredients: Snow pear 800 g, Sichuan scallops (Chuanbei) 10g, and rock sugar 10g.

Methods: Peel and core the snow pears, put these snow pears, Sichuan scallops and rock sugar into a bowl, and then simmer them for about 1 hour.

Actions: Moistening the lung and stopping cough.

Indicated population: People suffering from dry cough without phlegm and chronic cough.

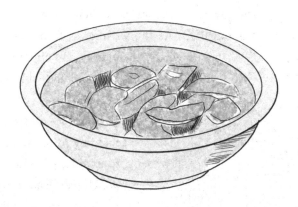

秋季 AUTUMN

霜降 First Frost (Shuangjiang)

霜降为每年公历 10 月 24 日前后，太阳黄经为 210°。霜降是秋季的最后一个节气，天气已冷，也意味着冬天即将到来。

In the Gregorian calendar, *First Frost* (Shuangjiang) usually begins around October 24th when the sun reaches the celestial longitude of 210°, which is the last solar term in autumn. It is cold in this solar term, which indicates the coming winter.

【霜降养生三妙招】Three hacks for health nurturing

❶ 防寒保暖

霜降节气最低气温可达 0℃左右，气候由凉转冷，此时要注意防寒保暖，尤其是易感冒、体质较弱的老年人和小儿，应适时增添衣物，以免寒风入侵，导致生病。除此之外，呼吸系统疾病患者防寒重点部位在背部，要注意背部的保暖；心脑血管系统疾病患者除了每日监测血压、按时服药外，不要盲目追求"秋冻"。

❶ Preventing cold and keeping warm

The lowest temperature of First Frost can be as low as about 0 ℃. As the weather is from cool to cold, we, especially the elderly and children who are easy to catch a cold and with weak constitution, should prevent cold and keep warm by adding clothes according to the weather so as to avoid cold wind invasion which may lead to illness. In addition, patients with respiratory diseases should focus on the back warmth; Except daily blood pressure monitoring and timely medication, patients with cardiovascular and cerebrovascular diseases should change into warmer clothes as soon as necessary.

❷ 动静结合

霜降后，气温越来越低，最好等太阳出来后出门锻炼，每次运动前，一定要做好充分的准备活动，注意动与静的合理结合。

❷ Appropriate exercise and rest

After *First Frost*, the temperature is getting lower and lower. It's better to go out for exercise after the sun comes out. Before exercising, be sure to make full preparations and combine exercise and rest appropriately.

❸ 饮食调理

霜降寒凉又干燥，胃肠道对寒冷的刺激非常敏感，可多吃芝麻、蜂蜜、银耳、青菜等食物，以及苹果、葡萄、香蕉等水果。

❸Dietary recommendation

It is cold and dry in First Frost. As the gastrointestinal tract tends to be very sensitive to cold stimulation, it is better to eat more sesame, honey, snow fungus, vegetables, as well as apples, grapes, bananas and other fruits.

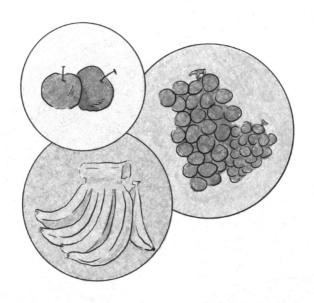

【霜降养生食疗方：栗子粥】

材料：栗子 150g，小米 200g。

做法：武火煮沸米粥后，用文火开盖继续煮 10 分钟；将栗子捣碎放入锅里，继续煮 5 分钟即可。

功效：补肾健脾，止泻治咳。

适宜人群：反复反胃、久咳、腹泻、腰膝酸软、骨折后期恢复者。

Health-nurturing recipe: Chestnut Porridge

Ingredients: Chestnut 150g and millet 200g.

Methods: After boiling the porridge with strong fire, open the lid and simmer for 10 minutes; Mash the chestnuts, put them into the pot and simmer for another 5 minutes.

Actions: Tonifying the kidney, strengthening the spleen, stopping diarrhea and relieving cough.

Indicated population: People with recurrent nausea, chronic cough, diarrhea, soreness and weakness of the waist and knees, and people who are recovering from fracture.

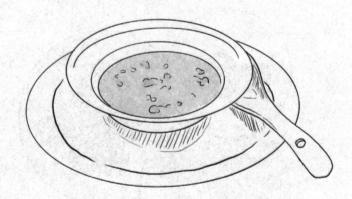

冬季 WINTER

　　冬三月，始于立冬，止于立春前，冬季分为立冬、小雪、大雪、冬至、小寒、大寒六个节气。

　　冬季是秋季和春季的过渡季节，我国南方为亚热带季风气候，冬季温和少雨；北方为温带季风气候，冬季寒冷干燥。

　　冬季天气寒冷，机体抵抗力下降，要早睡晚起，坚持温水刷牙、冷水洗脸、热水泡脚。

　　There are three months in winter, starting with *Beginning of Winter* (Lidong) and ending before *Beginning of Spring*, divided into six solar terms of *Beginning of Winter*, *Light Snow* (Xiaoxue), *Heavy Snow* (Daxue), *Winter Solstice* (Dongzhi), *Lesser Cold* (Xiaohan) and *Greater Cold* (Dahan).

　　Winter is the transitional period between autumn and spring. As for southern China, there is a subtropical monsoon climate which is mild and with little rain in winter; As for northern China, there is a temperate monsoon climate with cold and dry winters.

　　Due to the cold weather and decreased resistance, it is better to go to bed early and get up late. In addition, adhere to brush teeth with warm water, wash face with cold water, and soak feet with hot water.

宜：性味甘温的食物，如韭菜、茴香、姜、葱、蒜、鸡肉、羊肉、猪肝等。

Recommended: Sweet-flavored and warm-natured food, such as Chinese chives, fennel, ginger, green onion, garlic, chicken, mutton, pork liver, etc.

不宜：寒性食物，如苦瓜、竹笋、甘蔗、梨、西瓜、柿子、香蕉等。

Not recommended: Cold-natured food, such as bitter gourd, bamboo shoot, sugarcane, pear, watermelon, persimmon, banana, etc.

饮食

【食物足量，抵御寒冷】

冬季天寒地冻，机体在寒冷的环境中代谢率明显增加，人体对能量的需求也随之增加，需要保证足够量的主食，建议每天吃 250 ～ 400g 的主食，如米饭、馒头等。另外，每天应食用 150 ～ 250g 动物性食物，如瘦肉、鱼等，可提高抗寒防病的能力。

Enough food to resist the cold

In cold winter, the body's metabolic rate increases significantly in the cold environment, and the body's demand for energy increases accordingly. Thus, it is necessary to ensure sufficient intake of carbohydrates. It is suggested to eat 250-400 grams of carbos every day, such as rice, steamed bread, etc. In addition, 150-250 grams of meat, such as lean meat, fish, etc., should be taken every day to strengthen the immune system.

【少食生冷，多喝粥汤】

冬季食用生冷食物，容易刺激肠胃，造成腹痛、腹泻等。在制作冬季食物时，尽量多采用炖、煮、蒸、烩等烹调方式，多喝粥汤。

Less raw or cold food, more porridges and soups

Eating raw and cold food in winter can easily stimulate the stomach and intestines, resulting in abdominal pain, diarrhea and so on. When cooking in winter, try to use stewing, boiling, steaming, braising or other cooking methods. It is better to drink more porridges and soups.

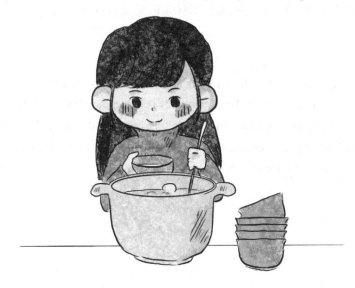

【多吃蔬果，预防干燥】

冬季干燥，容易出现便秘，应注意蔬菜水果的补充。蔬菜可选择萝卜、大白菜、马铃薯、山药、莲藕、香菇、冬笋、娃娃菜等，水果可选择苹果、梨、香蕉、柚子、柑橘等。

More fruits and vegetables to prevent dryness

Winter is dry and it is easy to cause constipation, so attention should be paid to the supplement of vegetables and fruits. As for vegetables, it is better to eat radish, Chinese cabbage, potato, yam, lotus root, shiitake, winter bamboo shoots, baby cabbage, etc.; As for fruits, it is better to eat apple, pear, banana, pomelo, citrus, etc.

【适量补充，点到为止】

冬季寒冷，日照时间缩短，户外活动少的人群，易导致维生素D 的缺乏，可多吃富含钙和维生素 D 的食物，如豆制品、海产品及动物肝脏等，但不能暴饮暴食，以免加重肠胃负担。

Appropriate supplement

In cold winter, shorter sunshine time and less outdoor exercise are easy to cause vitamin D deficiency. It is recommended to eat more foods rich in calcium and vitamin D, such as bean products, seafood and animal liver, but overeating is not allowed so as not to increase the burden of stomach and intestines.

睡眠

【早睡晚起】

冬季早睡晚起可避免低温和冷空气对人体入侵而诱发呼吸系统疾病，也可预防因严寒刺激诱发的心脑血管疾病。

Going to bed early and getting up late

Going to bed early and getting up late in winter can avoid the respiratory diseases due to invasion of cold air to human body, and can also prevent cardiovascular and cerebrovascular diseases induced by severe cold stimulation.

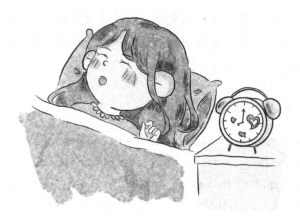

【 不要门窗紧闭 】

因冬季天气寒冷，人们常在睡觉时关上门窗，以致于空气不流通，易患感冒、咽炎等。建议睡觉时门窗保留一定缝隙，保持空气流通。

Avoiding closed doors and windows

Because of the cold weather in winter, people often close doors and windows when they sleep, so that the air does not circulate, and they are susceptible to colds and pharyngitis. It is suggested that windows could stay open with a small gap when sleeping to keep the room ventilated.

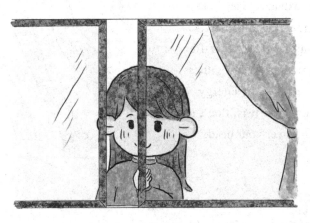

【别盖重棉被】

冬季盖厚重的被子会压迫胸部，影响正常呼吸，减少肺部的呼吸量，不仅影响睡眠，而且容易对呼吸道造成伤害。冬季应选用保暖松软的棉被、羽绒被等。

Avoiding heavy quilt

In winter, the thick and heavy quilt will compress the chest, affecting normal breathing, reducing the ventilation of the lungs, which not only affect sleep, but also easily cause injury to the respiratory tract. In winter, warm and soft quilt or duvet can be selected instead.

【不要蒙头睡】

蒙头睡觉，会因被窝内二氧化碳等废气逐渐增加，影响正常的呼吸。醒来后，易出现头晕、胸闷、乏力、精神不振。再冷的天气，睡眠时都不要用被子蒙头睡。

Don't sleep with head covered

Sleeping with your head covered will affect normal breathing due to the gradual increase of carbon dioxide and other exhaust gases in the space under the quilt. After waking up, it is easy to suffer from dizziness, chest tightness, fatigue and lack of energy. No matter how cold it is, don't sleep with a quilt over your head.

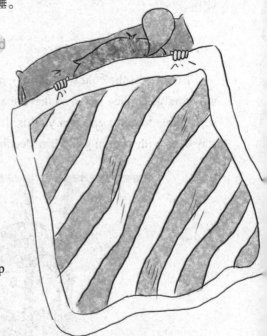

【不提倡裸睡】

冬季裸睡易受寒，且易引起头痛、目眩、咽喉肿痛等，因此不建议在冬季裸睡。

Avoiding naked sleep

Sleeping naked in winter is easy to lead to cold invasion which manifests as headache, dizziness, sore throat, etc., so it is not recommended.

活动

冬季活动，应选择在避风向阳、温暖安静、空气新鲜的旷野或有草坪之处，不要随意脱衣露体，尽量选择动作幅度较小、热量消耗较大的活动，活动时间控制在 1 个小时之内，推荐以下几项养生活动。

In winter, exercise should be done in the place where is no wind, sunny, warm, quiet and with fresh air and lawn. Maintain full coverage. It is better to choose exercises with less action range and high heat consumption and the time for exercise should be controlled within one hour. The following health-nurturing activities are recommended.

【冬泳】

冬泳能增强人体对冷刺激的适应能力，提高免疫力。建议每次游 100 ～ 500 米，下水前应做好热身运动。16 岁以下和 70 岁以上的人群，以及患有较为严重的心脏病、高血压、肝炎等疾病者，不宜冬泳。

Winter swimming

Winter swimming can enhance the adaptability of human body to cold stimulation and improve immunity. It is suggested to do a warm-up exercise before swimming and swim 100-500 meters every time. People under 16 years old and over 70 years old, as well as those with serious heart disease, high blood pressure, hepatitis and other diseases, are not suitable for winter swimming.

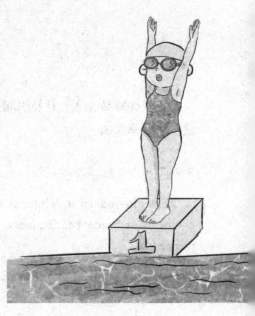

【滑雪】

滑雪可以锻炼身体的平衡能力、协调能力和柔韧性，对头、颈、手、腕、肘、臂、肩、腰、腿、膝、踝等部位能起到锻炼作用，建议每次滑雪1小时。患有心脏病、高血压、骨质疏松症等疾病，或做过大型手术者不宜滑雪。

Skiing

Skiing can improve the ability of balance, coordination and flexibility, and exercise the head, neck, hands, wrists, elbows, arms, shoulders, waist, legs, knees, ankles and other body parts. It is recommended to ski one hour each time. People suffering from heart disease, hypertension, osteoporosis and other diseases, or those who have had major surgeries should not ski.

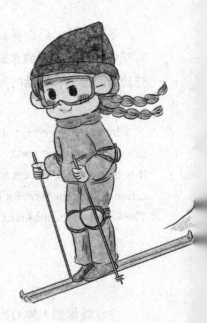

【跳绳】

冬季在室内跳绳是一个不错的选择。跳绳具有耗时少、耗能大的优点，还能增强人体心血管、呼吸和神经系统的功能。建议每次持续跳绳 10 分钟。老年人、骨质疏松、静脉曲张、膝盖旧伤未愈及体重过重者不宜跳绳。

Jump rope

In winter, jumping rope in-doors is a good choice with the advantages of less time and high energy consumption. In addition, it also can enhance the function of cardiovascular, respiratory and nervous system. It is recommended to jump rope for continuous 10 minutes each time. The elderly, people with osteoporosis, varicose veins and old knee injury and overweight people should not jump rope.

【泡温泉】

冬季泡温泉不仅可以促进身体的血液循环，还有助于纾解情绪压力、改善睡眠质量。建议每次泡温泉的时间不超过 15 分钟，温度不要超过 45℃。女性经期、孕妇、糖尿病患者、高血压患者不适宜此项活动。

Hot spring

Soaking in a hot spring in winter can not only promote blood circulation, but also relieve stress and improve sleep quality. It is recommended that each hot spring bath last no more than 15 minutes and the temperature should not exceed 45℃. It is not suitable for women with menstruation, pregnancy, diabetes, or hypertension.

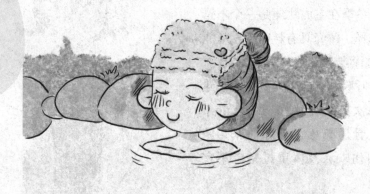

穴位养生

中医提倡冬养肾，因此应季养肾尤为重要。

Traditional Chinese medicine advocates nourishing the kidney in winter, so it is particularly important to nourish the kidney in season.

涌泉穴

【位置】脚掌上 1/3 正中位置的凹陷处。

【功效】温补肾阳。

【方法】每日晚上热水泡完脚后，用左手的大拇指点按右脚心上的涌泉穴约 100 次，左侧亦然。

Yongquan (KI 1)

Location: In the depression of the sole, which is approximately at the junction of the anterior 1/3 and posterior 2/3 of the sole.

Actions: Tonifying warmly the kidney yang.

Methods: After soaking feet in hot water every night, press Yongquan on the right foot with the left thumb for about 100 times, so does the left side.

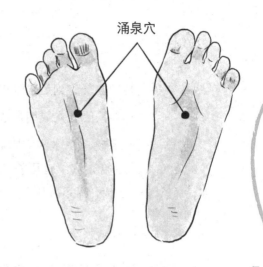

涌泉穴

气海穴

【位置】肚脐中间往下约两个横指的位置。

【功效】强壮体质。

【方法】将艾炷置于气海穴上，以有温热感为度，每次 5 ～ 7 壮，亦可采用艾条灸的方法，每次 10 ～ 20 分钟；还可以每天按揉此穴，以有酸胀感为宜。

Qihai (CV 6)

Location: About two fingers down from the middle of the navel.

Actions: Strengthening the body.

Methods: Place the moxa cone on Qihai for 5 to 7 cones each time, or moxibustion with moxa sticks for 10 to 20 min-

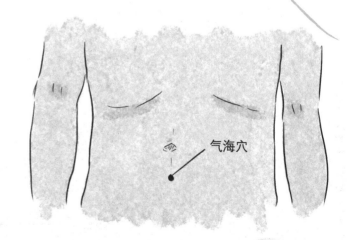

气海穴

utes is recommended, until warmth is felt; You can also press and rub this point every day until there is a sense of soreness and swelling.

太溪穴

【位置】足的内踝尖到足跟腱正中间凹陷处。

【功效】经常按摩此穴或用灸法，可提高免疫力。

【方法】每天晚上热水泡完脚后，用左手大拇指点按右侧太溪穴约 100 次，左侧亦然。也可将艾炷置于气海穴上，有温热感为度，每次 5 ～ 7 壮，还可采用艾条灸的方法，每次 10 ～ 20 分钟。

Taixi (KI 3)

Location: The depression from the tip of the inner ankle to the middle of the Achilles tendon of the foot.

Actions: Improving immunity by massage or moxibustion on this point.

Methods: After soaking feet in hot water every night, press Taixi on the right foot with the left thumb for about 100 times, so does the left side. Or place the moxa cone on Qihai for 5 to 7 cones each time or moxibustion with moxa sticks for 10 to 20 minutes is recommended, until there is warmth.

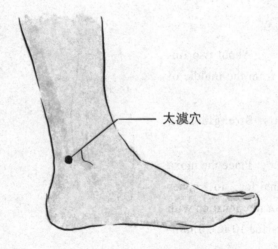

太溪穴

立冬 Beginning of Winter (Lidong)

立冬为每年公历 11 月 8 日前后，太阳黄经为 225°。立冬后，随着冷空气的加强，气温下降的趋势加快。

In the Gregorian calendar, *Beginning of Winter* (Lidong) usually begins around November 8th when the sun reaches the celestial longitude of 225°. After Beginning of Winter, the temperature drops quickly as the cold air intensifies.

【立冬养生应养肾】

立冬是冬天的开始，应以保养肾脏为先。

Nourishing the kidney for health nurturing

The first priority should be to nourish the kidney in *Beginning of Winter*.

❶ 推拿腰部

常常按揉或叩击腰骶部，摩擦腰部两侧，早晚各一次。平常漫步时，用双手背按揉肾区，可减缓腰酸。

❶ Massaging the waist

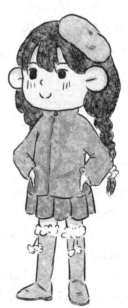

Frequently massage or tap the lumbosacral area and rub both sides of the waist in the morning and evening. When strolling, massaging the kidney area with the back of both hands can relieve lumbago.

❷ 护脚保暖

"脚暖腿不凉，腿暖身不寒"，寒从脚下起。脚步容易受到寒冷气息的影响，应穿保暖的鞋袜，护脚保暖。

❷Keeping feet warm

"Warm feet, no cold legs; Warm legs, no cold body". Cold usually invades the body from feet which are easily affected by the cold, so it is better to wear warm shoes and socks to keep feet warm.

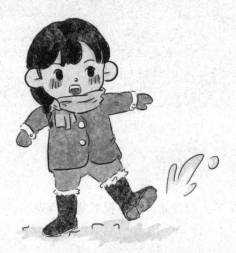

❸泡脚温肾

俗话说："热水洗脚，胜吃补药。"泡脚、按摩双脚能改善全身血液循环，达到滋养肾和肝的目的，每次泡脚时间以 30 ～ 45 分钟为宜，水温控制在 38 ～ 43℃，水要淹过脚踝，泡脚用的容器以木盆为宜。

❸Soaking feet to warm the kidney

As the saying goes, "Soaking feet in hot water is better than taking tonics." Soaking and massaging feet can improve blood circulation throughout the body to nourish the kidney and liver. It is suitable to soak feet in a wooden basin for 30 to 45 minutes each time, in the water of 38 to 43 ℃. The water should be over the ankles.

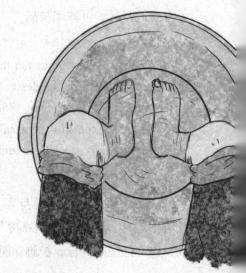

【立冬食疗方：十全大补汤】

材料：党参、黄芪、白术、茯苓、熟地、白芍各 10g，当归、肉桂各 5g，川芎、甘草各 3g，大枣 12 枚，生姜 20g，墨鱼、肥母鸡、老鸭、猪肚、肘子各 250g，排骨 500g，冬笋、蘑菇、花生、葱各 50g，黄酒、花椒、盐、味精适量。

做法：将诸药装纱布袋内，扎口，鸭、鸡肉及猪肚洗净，排骨剁开。生姜、冬笋、蘑菇洗净，与以上诸料同放锅中，加水，武火煮开后改用文火煨炖，加黄酒、花椒、盐调味。待肉熟烂后捞出，切成丝条，再放入汤内，去药袋，煮开后，调入味精，食肉饮汤。每次一小碗，早晚服用。

功效：温补气血，调五脏六腑。

适宜人群：神疲乏力、不进饮食、手脚无力、四肢关节疼痛者。

Health-nurturing recipe: Ten Powerful Tonics Decoction

Ingredients: Tangshen (Dangshen), astragalus, largehead atractylodes rhizome (Baizhu), indian bread (Fuling), prepared rehmannia root (Shudi) and debark peony root (Baishao) each 10g; Chinese angelica (Danggui) and cassia bark (Rougui) each 5g; Sichuan lovage rhizome (Chuanxiong) and liquorice each 3g; 12 jujubes; fresh ginger 20g; cuttlefish, poulard, old duck, pork tripe and ham hock each 250g; pork ribs 500g; winter bamboo shoots, mushrooms, peanut and green onion each 50g; appropriate amount of yellow rice wine, Sichuan pepper, salt and MSG.

Methods: Put the medicine into a gauze bag, tie the bag, wash the duck, chicken, pork tripe, fresh ginger, winter bamboo shoots and mushrooms, chop the ribs, and then put the above ingredients together in the pot. Add water, bring them to a boil over strong fire, and then simmer them, adding yellow rice wine, Sichuan pepper and salt. When these meats are rotten, bring them out to cut them into strips, and then put them back and remove the bag. After boiling, add appropriate amount of MSG. And then it's ready. Take one small bowl each time in the morning and evening.

Actions: Tonifying warmly qi and blood and regulating five *zang*-organs and six *fu*-organs.

Indicated population: People with fatigue, lack of strength, poor appetite, hand and foot weakness, and joint pain.

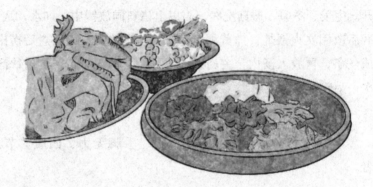

小雪 Light Snow (Xiaoxue)

小雪为每年公历 11 月 23 日前后，太阳黄经为 240°。气温下降，开始降雪，但还不到大雪纷飞的时节，故称小雪。小雪前后，黄河流域开始降雪，北方已进入封冻季节。

In the Gregorian calendar, *Light Snow* (Xiaoxue) usually begins around November 23rd when the sun reaches the celestial longitude of 240°. As the temperature drops, it begins to snow, but it is not yet the time for heavy snow, so this solar term is called *Light Snow*. Around *Light Snow*, snow begins to fall in the Yellow River basin, and the northern China has entered the freezing season.

【小雪注意防冻疮】

小雪起，天气湿冷，皮肤局部小动脉发生收缩，久之动脉血管麻痹而扩张，静脉瘀血、局部血液循环不良而致使冻疮高发。

Preventing frostbite

From *Light Snow*, with the cold and wet weather, the local arterioles contract, resulting in dilated arteries due to paralysis, venous blood stasis and local poor blood circulation, which lead to a high incidence of frostbite.

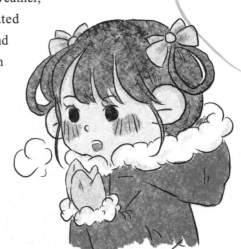

❶ 揉搓防冻

每天数次揉搓手、耳等局部皮肤，每次数分钟至局部皮肤发热为止，用揉搓的方法加强局部的摩擦，以迅速改善局部的血液循环，防止冻伤。

❶ Preventing frostbite by rubbing

Rub hands, ears and other local skin for several

minutes each time until the local skin is hot, several times a day, which can strengthen the local friction, so as to quickly improve the local blood circulation to prevent frostbite.

❷ 防寒保暖

应注意身体局部的保暖，尤其是裸露在外的身体部位，如耳朵可戴耳罩、双手可戴保暖手套、双脚穿保暖袜。

❷Keeping warm

Attention should be paid to the local warmth of the body, especially the exposed body parts, such as earmuffs for the ears, warm gloves for the hands, and warm socks for the feet.

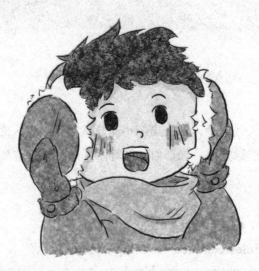

❸ 中药外泡

使用中药外泡，可预防冻疮。如当归四逆汤，即取当归、芍药、桂枝、细辛、甘草、木通、生姜、大枣煮水，外泡手足易患冻疮部位，水温控制在40℃左右，每次泡20分钟。

❸Soaking with Chinese medicine

Soaking with Chinese medicine can prevent frostbite, such as Chinese Angelica Frigid Extremities Decoction (Danggui Sini Tang) which is boiled by Chinese angelica, Chinese peony (Shaoyao), cassia twig (Guizhi), manchurian wildginger root (Xixin), licorice, akebia stem (Mutong), fresh ginger and jujube. Hands and feet which is vulnerable to frostbite can be soaked in this decoction for 20 minutes each time, and control the water temperature at around 40 ℃.

【小雪食疗方：黄芪桂圆牛肉汤】

材料：黄芪 10g，桂圆肉 20g，牛肉 200g，豌豆苗 20g，盐 3g，白酒 2g。

做法：牛肉切片，加水 1500mL 同煮，煮沸后去除泡沫及油。加入黄芪及桂圆肉，煮至水余约 600mL 为止，加盐、白酒调味，再加入豌豆苗，滚熟即成。

功效：补心安神，强筋壮骨。

适宜人群：食欲不振、消瘦乏力、体虚出汗、面色萎黄、失眠健忘、心中烦躁者。

Health-nurturing recipe: Stewed Beef with Astragalus and Longan

Ingredients: Astragalus 10g, longan 20g, beef 200g, pea sprout 20g, salt 3g and Chinese baijiu 2g.

Methods: Slice the beef and add 1500 mL of water to boil. Skim the foam and oil after boiling. Add astragalus and longan, boil until about 600 mL of water remains, add salt, Chinese baijiu and pea sprouts, and then it's ready when they are cooked.

Actions: Tonifying the heart, tranquilizing mind and strengthening the tendon and bones.

Indicated population: People with poor appetite, emaciation, lack of strength, weakness, sweating, sallow complexion, insomnia, forgetfulness and irritability.

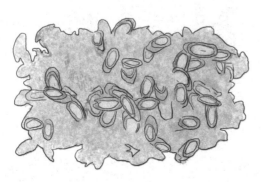

大雪 Heavy Snow (Daxue)

大雪为每年公历 12 月 7 日前后，太阳黄经为 255°。大雪节气，预示冬季最寒冷的时候到了，这时我国大部分地区的最低温度都降到了 0℃或以下，往往在北方会降大雪，甚至暴雪。

In the Gregorian calendar, *Heavy Snow* (Daxue) usually begins around December 7th when the sun reaches the celestial longitude of 255°. This solar term heralds the arrival of the coldest time of winter, when the minimum temperature in most parts of China falls to 0℃ or below, often with heavy snowfall or even blizzards in the north.

【大雪防风寒感冒】
Preventing common cold due to wind cold in Heavy Snow

❶ 多喝热水

每天饮水量不少于 2000mL，保证身体的水分充足，有利于身体排毒，预防感冒，但要多喝热水，少喝冷水。

❶ Drinking more hot water

Drink not less than 2,000 mL of water a day to ensure that the body is well hydrated, which is conducive to detoxification of the body and prevention of colds, but drink more hot water and less cold water.

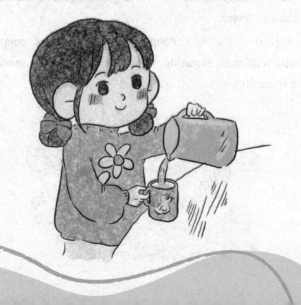

❷ 荤素搭配

冬季是进补的季节，在进补时需格外注意饮食的荤素搭配，多吃蔬菜水果，如大白菜、萝卜、香蕉、梨和苹果等，少吃油腻、辛辣食物。

❷Appropriate meat and vegetables

Winter is the season of tonic. At this time, we should balance the intake of meat and vegetable in our diet. Eat more vegetables and fruits, such as cabbage, radish, bananas, pears and apples, etc., and eat less greasy and spicy food.

❸ 全身保暖

大雪节气，稍不注意就会受风寒而患上感冒，除了要穿上厚毛衣、羽绒服、保暖裤外，还要做好头部、颈部及脚部等部位的保暖工作。

❸Keeping the whole body warm

In this solar term, a little carelessness may lead to colds due to wind cold. We should not only wear thick sweaters, down jackets and thermal pants, but also keep warm in the head, neck and feet.

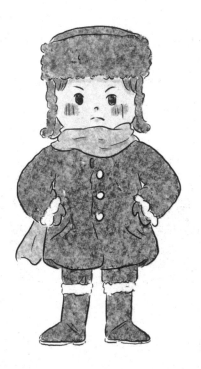

【大雪食疗方：蒜泥茼蒿】

材料：茼蒿 250g，大蒜 3 瓣，味精、盐、香油适量。

做法：茼蒿洗净，切一寸长段，大蒜捣烂为泥备用，锅内放入清水煮开，茼蒿下锅焯 3 分钟捞出，将蒜泥、味精、盐、香油同时放入，搅拌均匀盛盘即可。

功效：开胃健脾，解毒消积。

适宜人群：腹胀不思饮食、口淡无味者。

Health-nurturing recipe: Mixed Mashed Garlic and Crown Daisy

Ingredients: Crown daisy 250g, 3 cloves of garlic, and appropriate amount of MSG, salt and sesame oil.

Methods: Wash the crown daisy and cut it into one-inch-long pieces. Mash the garlic into puree and set it aside. Bring clean water to a boil in the pot. Blanch the crown daisy for 3 minutes and take it out. Add the mashed garlic, MSG, salt and sesame oil at the same time. Mix them well and serve.

Actions: Stimulating appetite, strengthening the spleen, resolving toxin and stagnation.

Indicated population: People with abdominal distension, poor appetite and tastelessness.

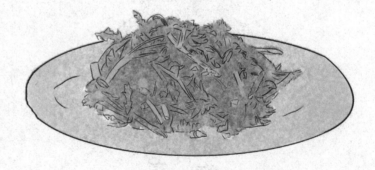

冬至 Winter Solstice (Dongzhi)

冬至为每年公历 12 月 22 日前后，太阳黄经为 270°。冬至这一天，阳光几乎直射南回归线，北半球白昼最短，黑夜最长，开始进入数九寒天。而冬至以后，阳光直射位置逐渐向北移动，北半球白天就逐渐长了。

In the Gregorian calendar, *Winter Solstice* (Dongzhi) usually begins around December 22nd when the sun reaches the celestial longitude of 270°. On Winter Solstice, the direct sunlight is on the Tropic of Capricorn, which indicates the shortest day and longest night in the northern hemisphere and also the beginning of the coldest days. After *Winter Solstice*, the position of direct sunlight gradually moves northward, which indicates that the days in the northern hemisphere gradually lengthen.

【冬至吃羊肉】Eating mutton

❶ 羊肉并非人人适宜

羊肉既能御风寒，又可补身体，但并非人人适宜，如经常口舌糜烂、眼睛发红、口苦、烦躁、咽喉干痛、牙龈肿痛、腹泻者均忌吃羊肉。

❶ Mutton, not suitable for everyone

Mutton can not only protect against wind cold, but also can supplement the body, however, it is not suitable for everyone. People who often suffer from mouth erosion, red eyes, bitter mouth, irritability, sore throat, swollen gums and diarrhea should not eat mutton.

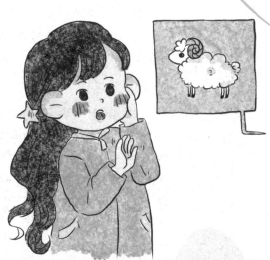

❷ 羊肉炖吃最营养

羊肉经过炖制以后，更加熟烂、鲜嫩，易于消化。如果在炖的时候加上合适的中药（甘草、当归、生姜、桂皮、八角等），更具进补功效。

❷Stewing, the most nutritious methods for cooking mutton

After stewing, mutton is more cooked, tender and easy to digest. If you add appropriate Chinese medicine (licorice, Chinese angelica, fresh ginger, cinnamon, star anise, etc.) when stewing, it will have tonic effect.

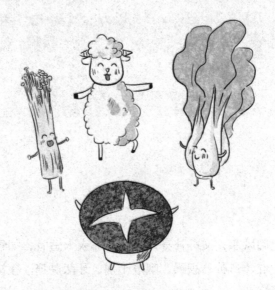

❸ 合理搭配防上火

羊肉性温热，常吃容易上火。因此，吃羊肉时要搭配凉性和甘平性的蔬菜，如冬瓜、丝瓜、菠菜、白菜、金针菇、蘑菇、冬笋等。

❸Reasonable coordination to prevent fire

Mutton is warm and hot in property, which is easy to cause excessive internal heat. Therefore, when eating mutton, it is necessary to coordinate with cool-naturedand sweet-neutral vegetables, such as white gourd, sponge gourd, spinach, Chinese cabbage, enokitake, mushrooms, winter bamboo shoots, etc.

❹吃羊肉时忌醋、茶

羊肉大热，醋性甘温，有开胃、活血、杀菌等作用，羊肉中含有蛋白质、糖类、维生素和多种有机酸，同食不仅会削弱羊肉的食疗作用，而且会对人体有害。另外，吃羊肉时或吃完羊肉马上饮茶，会减弱肠蠕动，减少大便中的水分，而引起便秘。

❹Avoiding vinegar and tea when eating mutton

Mutton is extreme hot in property. However, vinegar is sweet and warm in property, which can stimulate appetite, promote blood circulation and sterilize. Mutton contains protein, carbohydrate, vitamins and a variety of organic acids. The combination of these two will not only weaken the therapeutic effect of mutton, but also be harmful to human body. In addition, drinking tea immediately when eating mutton or after eating mutton will weaken intestinal peristalsis, reduce the water in stool, and lead to constipation.

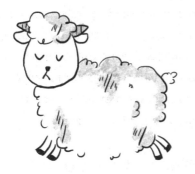 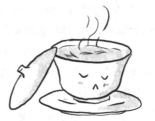

❺羊肉虽好应适量

羊肉富含蛋白质和脂肪，但过多食用会影响肝脏的功能，从而加重肝病患者的病情。

❺Mutton, moderate intake recommended

Mutton is rich in protein and fat, but eating too much will affect the liver function, thus aggravating the condition of patients with liver disease.

【冬至食疗方：白萝卜炖羊肉】

材料： 白萝卜 200g，羊肉 200g，葱、姜、花椒适量。

做法： 羊肉切块于沸水中去血水后，于凉水中上锅煮，火开后关火，将羊肉捞出，冲掉血沫。葱切段，姜切片，与花椒、羊肉一起置锅中煮。白萝卜洗净切成块，放于锅中，盖上锅盖，武火煮至水开，换中文火煮 1.5 小时。

功效： 温阳祛寒，补气益血。

适宜人群： 腰膝酸软，形瘦怕冷，小便不畅，病后体虚、怕冷，产妇产后出血或腹痛者。

Health-nurturing recipe: Stewed Mutton with Daikon

Ingredients: Daikon 200g, mutton 200g, and appropriate amount of green onion, ginger and Sichuan pepper.

Methods: Cut the mutton into pieces in boiling water, remove the water with blood, boil them in cold water, turn off the fire after boiling, fish out the mutton and wash away the blood foam. Cut the green onion into sections, slice the ginger, and cook mutton with Sichuan pepper and them. Wash the daikon and cut it into pieces, put them in a pot and cover the pot. Boil the water with strong fire and turn to gentle fire for 1.5 hours after boiling.

Actions: Warming yang, repelling cold, tonifying qi and boosting blood.

Indicated population: People with soreness and weakness of the waist and knees, emaciation, afraid of cold, poor urination, deficiency after disease, postpartum hemorrhage or abdominal pain.

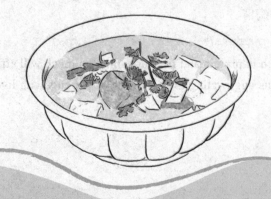

小寒 Lesser Cold (Xiaohan)

小寒为每年公历 1 月 6 日前后，太阳黄经为 285°。小寒以后，气温急剧下降，冷气积久而寒，标志着一年中最寒冷的日子就要到来了。

In the Gregorian calendar, *Lesser Cold* (Xiaohan) usually begins around January 6th when the sun reaches the celestial longitude of 285°. After *Lesser Cold*, the temperature drops sharply, the cold air accumulates for a long time and becomes colder, marking the arrival of the coldest day of the year.

【小寒养生做好"三防""四补"】
"Three Preventions and Four Tonifying" for health nurturing

❶ "三防"

一防头颈寒：小寒时节，保暖是第一要务，尤其要注意头颈部保暖，外出记得穿高领衣服，戴围脖、帽子等保护头颈。

❶ "Three Preventions"

First, preventing head and neck against cold. During Lesser Cold, keeping warm is the first priority, especially in the head and neck. When going out, remember to wear high-collared clothes, scarves, hats to protect the head and neck.

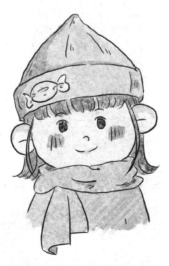

冬季 WINTER

135

二防身受凉：腹部是连接身体上下的枢纽，人体身上很多重要的穴位都在腹部，如神阙、气海、关元等。腹部保暖除了平时要保证穿着外，也可两手搓热后进行按摩。

Second, prevent the body against cold. The abdomen connects the upper and lower parts of the body and there are many important acupoints, such as Shenque (CV 8), Qihai, Guanyuan (ST 22), etc. In addition to usual wearing, massaging with warm hands can also keep abdomen warm.

三防脚不暖：除了穿保暖的鞋子外，最好睡前用热水泡脚，然后用力揉搓脚心，促进血液循环。

Three, keeping feet warm. In addition to wearing warm shoes, it is best to use hot water to soak your feet before going to bed, and then rub the soles of feet hard to promote blood circulation.

❷ "四补"

一补气：易冒虚汗、易疲乏、身体虚弱者等人群宜用红参、红枣、白术、北黄芪、山药、五味子等补气，泡水或炖肉食用均可。

❷"Four Tonifying"

First, tonifying qi. Red ginseng (Hongshen), jujube, largehead atractylodes rhizome, astragalus, Henan yam and chinese magnoliavine fruit (Wuweizi), soaked in the water or stewed with meat, are suitable to tonify qi for people with sweating due to deficiency, fatigue and weakness.

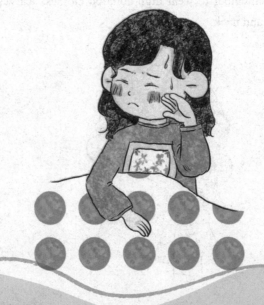

二补血：头昏眼花、面色苍白等人群宜用当归、熟地黄、白芍和首乌等补血，泡水或炖肉食用均可。

Second, tonifying blood. Chinese angelica, prepared rehmannia root, debark peony root and fleeceflower root (Shouwu), soaked in the water or stewed with meat, are suitable to tonify blood for people with dizziness and pale complexion.

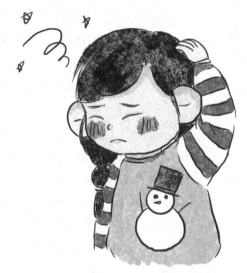

三补阴：夜间汗多、手足心热等人群宜用冬虫夏草、白参、沙参、天冬、白木耳等补阴，泡水或炖肉食用均可。

Three, tonifying yin. Chinese caterpillar fungus (Dongchongxiacao), white ginseng (Baishen), asparagus (Tiandong) and snow fungus, soaked in the water or stewed with meat, are suitable to tonify yin for people with sweating at night, feverish sensation in the soles of hands and feet.

四补阳：手足冰凉、腰酸怕冷等人群宜炖服核桃、栗子，或用韭菜、茴香等泡水或炖服均可。

Four, tonifying yang. Stewing walnuts and chestnuts, or soaking or stewing Chinese chives and fennel is suitable for people who has cold hands and feet, soreness in the waist and are fear of cold.

【 小寒食疗方：当归生姜羊肉汤 】

材料：当归 20g，生姜 30g，羊肉 500g，黄酒、调料适量。

做法：将羊肉洗净，切为碎块，加入当归、生姜、黄酒及调料，炖煮 1 ～ 2 小时，食肉喝汤。

功效：健脾补血，祛寒强身。

适宜人群：腹胀冷痛，手足冰冷，体虚所致的月经不调、痛经，风湿关节炎，跌打损伤之机体疼痛不适，体虚怕冷者。

Health-nurturing recipe: Stewed Mutton with Chinese Angelica and Ginger

Ingredients: Chinese angelica 20g, fresh ginger 30g, mutton 500g and appropriate amount of yellow rice wine and other condiments.

Methods: Wash the mutton, cut it into pieces, add Chinese angelica, fresh ginger, yellow rice wine and condiments, stew for 1 to 2 hours, and then eat meat and drink soup.

Actions: Strengthening the spleen, tonifying blood, expelling cold and strengthening body.

Indicated population: People with abdominal distension with cold pain, cold hands and feet, irregular menstruation and dysmenorrhea due to body deficiency, rheumatoid arthritis and pain due to traumatic injury; People who are fear of cold due to deficiency.

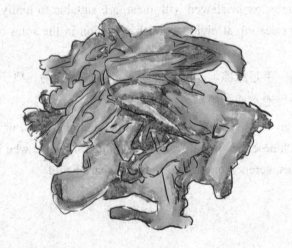

大寒 Greater Cold (Dahan)

大寒为每年公历 1 月 20 日前后，太阳黄经为 300°。大寒是全年二十四节气中的最后一个节气，在我国常出现大范围降温、大风、雨雪的天气，呈现出冰天雪地、天寒地冻的严寒景象。

In the Gregorian calendar, *Greater Cold* (Dahan) usually begins around January 20th when the sun reaches the celestial longitude of 300°, which is the last solar term. On this solar term, there is often widespread cooling, heavy wind, rain and snow, presenting a cold scene in China.

【大寒养生防三大系统疾病】
Preventing diseases of three systems for health nurturing

❶ 心脑血管系统疾病

大寒是中风、心肌梗死等疾病的发病高峰期。冷空气会刺激人体毛细血管的收缩，血管阻力增大，导致血压升高，心脏负荷加重，容易诱发冠心病等。寒冷还会引起冠状动脉痉挛，影响心脏血液供应，诱发心肌梗死等，所以大寒要做好预防心脑血管疾病的工作。

❶Cardiovascular and cerebrovascular diseases

Greater Cold is the peak period of stroke, myocardial infarction and other diseases, because cold air can stimulate the contraction of capillaries, increase vascular resistance, resulting in increased blood pressure and heart load, which are easy to induce coronary heart disease. In addition, cold can also cause coronary artery spasm, affecting the blood supply of the heart and inducing myocardial infarction, etc., so it is better to prevent cardiovascular and cerebrovascular diseases in *Greater Cold*.

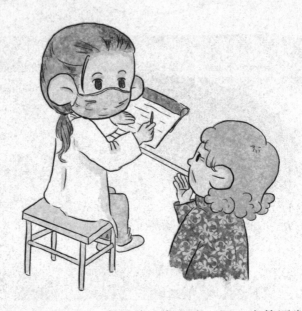

首先要做好高血压、高血糖、高血脂、冠心病等原发病的治疗；其次要注意防寒保暖，适当加强体育锻炼以促进气血畅和；睡前可用热水或生姜、艾叶、花椒、当归等中药煮水泡脚，可起到驱寒散湿、活血通络的作用。另外，要注意及时发现预兆症状，如有不适立即就近就医。

First of all, manage the primary diseases well including hypertension, hyperglycemia, hyperlipidemia, coronary heart disease and other diseases; Secondly, keep warm and take apropriate exercise to promote the smooth flow of qi and blood; Before going to bed, soak feet with hot water or boiling water of ginger, wormwood, Sichuan pepper, Chinese angelica and other Chinese medicine can dispel cold and dampness, promote blood circulation and dredge collaterals. In addition, pay attention to premonitory symptoms in time, and go to hospital nearby immediately if patients are discomfort.

❷ 呼吸系统疾病

大寒节气是一年中最冷的时期，气候干燥寒冷，此时人体的免疫力也随之下降，感冒、咽炎、支气管炎、肺气肿等呼吸系统疾病高发，尤其是孩子和老年人应格外注意。

❷ Respiratory diseases

Greater Cold is the coldest period in a year, with the dry and cold weather. At this time, the immunity also declines, so respiratory diseases often occur, such as colds, pharyngitis, bronchitis and emphysema. Children and the elderly should pay special attention to these diseases.

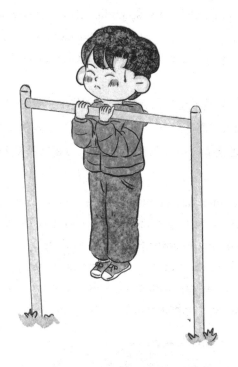

在寒冷的大寒节气要注意防寒保暖，尤其要重视对头颈部、胸腹部、腰背和四肢等容易受寒部位的保护。同时要适当进行体育锻炼以增强身体抵抗力，防止呼吸系统疾病发生。

During this cold solar term, pay attention to keep warm, especially head, neck, chest, abdomen, waist, back, limbs and other body parts which is vulnerable to cold. At the same time, it is better to take proper physical exercise to enhance the immunity to prevent respiratory diseases.

❸ 消化系统疾病

大寒节气，人体受寒冷刺激后血液中的组织胺增多，胃酸分泌旺盛，胃肠发生痉挛收缩，机体抗病能力及适应性也随之降低，故胃肠疾病易复发。同时因天气寒冷，人们多爱进补，大吃大喝也易伤了脾胃。

❸Digestive system diseases

During *Greater Cold*, after the cold stimulation, the histamine in the blood increases, the gastric acid secretes more, the gastrointestinal spasm occurs, and the immunity and adaptability also decrease, so the gastro-intestinal diseases are easy to relapse. At the same time, because of the cold weather, people eat and drink a lot, which is easy to hurt the spleen and stomach.

此时更应注意保养脾胃，防止消化系统疾病的发生。三餐定时，不暴饮暴食；慎进香辣、油炸肥腻食物；多食易消化的食物。同时要注意腹部保暖，可多做腹部按摩，必要时外敷热水袋或中药热敷包。

At this time, more attention should be paid to the maintenance of the spleen and stomach to prevent digestive system diseases. Eat three meals regularly, do not overeat; Be careful with spicy, fried and greasy food; Eat more digestible food. At the same time, pay attention to keep the abdomen warm by massaging the abdomen more, hot-water bag or Chinese medicine hot compress bag, if necessary.

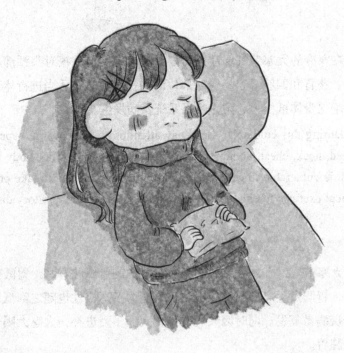

【大寒食疗方：黄芪枸杞炖童子鸡】

材料：童子鸡1只（约500g），黄芪30g，枸杞子30g，白术10g，盐适量。

做法：将童子鸡洗净，切成小块，加入黄芪、枸杞子、白术和盐，用文火慢炖1小时，食肉喝汤。

功效：调养脾胃，滋补肝肾。

适宜人群：腰膝酸软、潮热盗汗、眼睛干涩，或年老体虚、气虚怯冷者。

Health-nurturing recipe: Stewed Poussin with Astragalus and Chinese Wolfberry

Ingredients: One poussin (about 500g), astragalus 30g, Chinese wolfberry 30g, largehead atractylodes rhizome 10g, and appropriate amount of salt.

Methods: Wash the poussin, cut it into pieces, add astragalus, Chinese wolfberry, largehead atractylodes rhizome and salt, simmer for one hour, and then eat the meat and drink the soup.

Actions: Regulating the spleen and stomach, and nourishing and tonifying the liver and kidney.

Indicated population: People with soreness and weakness of the waist and knees, tidal fever, night sweating and dry eyes; Or the elderly who are weak and fear of cold due to qi deficiency.

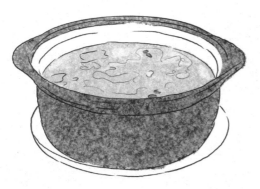

新型冠状病毒肺炎
防疫小知识
Novel Coronavirus
Pneumonia Prevention Tips

"宅"家自我健康管理方法
Self-health Management Methods at Home

2020 年初春，在抗击新型冠状病毒肺炎疫情中，中医药发挥了特色优势作用。编者根据新型冠状病毒肺炎防控的理论知识，结合防疫工作经验，提出了"宅"家自我健康管理方法。

In the early spring of 2020, TCM played a unique role in the fight against the novel coronavirus pneumonia. Based on theoretical knowledge of the prevention and control of novel coronavirus pneumonia and experience in epidemic prevention work, the editors propose a method of self-health management at home.

❶ 避毒抗疫，远离戾气

常开门窗，通风换气；正确洗手，加强消毒；做好防护，远离病毒。

❶Avoid viruses and epidemics, and stay away from pestilent qi

Open doors and windows often for ventilation; Wash hands properly and strengthen disinfection; Take care of protection to stay away from viruses.

❷ 起居有常，合理睡眠

夜卧早起，广步于庭；作息有时，适当午睡。

❷Have regular daily life and reasonable sleep

Sleep at night and get up early, and take a walk; Work and rest regularly, and take a nap properly.

❸ 饮食有节，平衡膳食

谷蛋肉奶，果蔬多样；五味调和，清淡营养；寒热温凉，切莫偏样；慎食生冷，远离野味；戒烟限酒，饮水莫忘。

❸Have a regular and balanced diet

Eat grain, egg, meat and milk, various fruits and vegetables; Five flavors are harmonious, and have a light and nutritious diet; Eat food in cold, hot, warm and cool, and don't be partial; Eat raw and cold food properly and stay away from wild food; Quit smoking, limit alcohol and don't forget to drink water.

❹ 调畅情志，心理健康

情志舒畅，修身养性；宁静致远，道法自然；笑口常开，和谐共处。

❹ Regulate emotions and mental health

Relax the emotion and spirit, cultivate yourself; Be tranquil to go far and follow the nature; Smile often, and live in harmony.

❺ 劳逸适度，科学运动

劳逸结合，不妄作劳；动静相宜，气血调和；合理用脑，益智防衰；科学运动，居家练习。

❺ Work and rest moderately, and exercise scientifically

Combine work and rest, and do not work recklessly; Be suitable for movement and static, harmony of qi and blood; Use brain rationally to improve the intelligence and prevent decline; Exercise scientifically at home.

❻ 推拿按摩，舒通经络

头面热搓，疏风开窍；后枕按揉，提神醒脑；饭后摩腹，益气健脾；睡前泡脚，揉足助眠。

❻ Massage and dredge the meridians

Rub the head and face until there is heat feeling to disperse wind and open the orifices; Massage the posterior occipital area to refresh your mind; Rub the abdomen after meals to boost qi and strengthen the spleen; Soak your feet before going to bed and rub your feet to help you sleep.

❼ 芳香辟秽，抗毒驱邪

湿浊热毒，疫戾从之；芳香之品，辟秽防瘟；香薰香囊，常备常用。

❼Ward off filth with aroma, avoid viruses and repel the evil

Pestilence comes from dampness, turbidity and heat toxin; Ward off filth and prevent pestilence with aromatic products; Prepare and use aromatherapy and sachet.

❽穴位艾灸，固护阳气

找准穴位，循经取穴；艾条温灸，温阳扶正；艾灸虽好，因人而异。

❽Moxibustion at acupoints with moxa to protect yang qi

Select acupoints along the meridian to find the right acupoints; Moxibustion with moxa, warm yang to reinforce healthy qi; although moxibustion is good, it varies from person to person.

❾及时就医，防微杜渐

慢性疾病，切莫停药；发热咳嗽，就近就医。

❾Seek medical attention in time to prevent at the beginning

For chronic diseases, do not stop the medication; if you have a fever or cough, seek medical attention nearby.

提高免疫力食疗方
Health-nurturing Recipe for Enhancing Immunity

中医理论认为，人体免疫力是预防疾病的第一道防线，而合理的营养膳食是改善个人营养状况和增强免疫力的重要因素。很多食材及中药具有提高人体免疫力的作用，对于免疫力较低的人群，可通过食补进行一定干预。

According to TCM theory, human immunity is the first line of defense against disease, and an appropriate nutritional diet is an important factor in improving one's nutritional condition and enhancing immunity. Many ingredients and herbs have the effect of improving human immunity, and for people with low immunity, interventions can be made through dietary supplements.

银耳枸杞汤 Snow Fungus and Chinese Wolfberry Soup

【材料】银耳 20g，枸杞子 15g，冰糖适量。

【做法】银耳泡发，撕碎成片，与枸杞子一同入锅，加适量清水，文火炖煮 20 分钟，加入适量冰糖，煮至冰糖溶化，即可食用。

【功效】养阴润肺，滋补肝肾。

【适宜人群】口干咽燥，干咳无痰，失眠健忘者。

Ingredients: Snow fungus 20g, Chinese wolfberry 15g, and appropriate amount of rock sugar.

Methods: Soak the snow fungus, shred the rehydrated snow fungus into pieces, put them into the pot with the Chinese wolfberry, add an appropriate amount of water, simmer for 20 minutes, add an appropriate amount of rock sugar, cook until the rock sugar melts before eating.

Actions: Nourishing yin to moisten the lung, and nourishing and tonifying the liver and kidney.

Indicated population: People with dry mouth and throat, dry cough without phlegm, insomnia and forgetfulness.

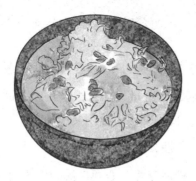

黄芪红枣茶 Astragalus and Jujube Tea

【材料】黄芪 30g，红枣 5 颗。

【做法】红枣用温水泡发洗净后，去核，黄芪用清水浸泡 20 分钟，两物加适量清水，煮沸后文火煮 20 分钟，当茶饮。

【功效】益气健脾，养血安神。

【适宜人群】身体虚弱，面色无华，乏力汗多者。

Ingredients: Astragalus 5 g, and 5 jujubes.

Methods: Soak jujubes in warm water, rinse the rehydrated jujubes and core them. Soak the astragalus in water for 20 minutes. Add an appropriate amount of water. After boiling, simmer for 20 minutes, and then drink as tea.

Actions: Boosting qi and strengthening the spleen, and nourishing the blood and calming the mind.

Indicated population: People with weak constitution, pale complexion, fatigue and profuse sweating.

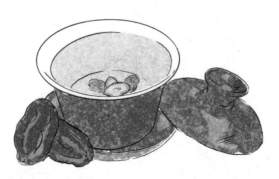

西洋参瘦肉粥 American ginseng and Lean meat Porridge

【材料】西洋参 10g（切片），瘦肉 250g，粳米 250g。

【做法】汤锅加水适量，加入洗净粳米，武火煮 5 分钟后，加入西洋参及瘦肉，待水开后，改用文火炖煮，半小时后即可食用。

【功效】补气养阴，健脾补肺。

【适宜人群】神疲乏力，心烦口渴，体虚消渴者。

Ingredients: American ginseng 10g (pieces), lean meat 250g and rice 250g.

Methods: Add an appropriate amount of water to the soup pot, add washed rice, cook over strong heat for 5 minutes, and add American ginseng and lean meat. After boiling, simmer for half an hour before eating.

Actions: Tonifying qi, nourishing yin, strengthening the spleen and tonifying the lung.

Indicated population: People with fatigue, vexation, thirst, weak constitution and diabetic.

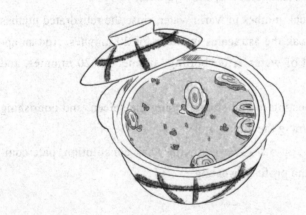

主要参考文献 References

董易奇. 中华万年历 [M]. 北京：中国工人出版社，2013.

Dong Yiqi. *Chinese Lunar Calender*[M]. Beijing: China workers Publishing House, 2013.

郭长青. 实用针灸经络穴位图谱 [M]. 上海：上海科学技术出版社，2013.

Guo Changqing. *Practical Illustrated Book of Meridians and Acupoints*[M]. Shanghai: Shanghai Scientific and Technical Publishers, 2013.

高鹏翔. 中医学 [M]. 北京：人民卫生出版社，2013.

Gao Pengxiang. *Traditional Chinese Medicine*[M]. Beijing: People's Medical Publishing House, 2013.

郭霞珍. 中医基础理论 [M]. 上海：上海科学技术出版社，2012.

Guo Xiazhen. *Basic Theory of Traditional Chinese Medicine*[M]. Shanghai: Shanghai Scientific and Technical Publishers, 2012.

钱超尘. 伤寒杂病论版本通鉴 [M]. 北京：北京科学技术出版社，2017.

Qian Chaochen. *A General Introduction to Versions of Shanghan Zabing Lun*[M]. Beijing: Beijing Science and Technology Publishing Co., Ltd., 2017.

曲黎敏. 养生十二说 [M]. 北京：中国对外翻译出版公司，2008.

Qu Limin. *Twelve Lessons on Health Nurturing*[M]. Beijing: China Translation Corporation, 2008.

孙广仁. 中医基础理论 [M]. 第二版. 北京：中国中医药出版社，2007.

Sun Guangren. *Basic Theory of Traditional Chinese Medicine* (2nd version) [M]. Beijing: China Press of Traditional Chinese Medicine, 2007.

徐文兵. 黄帝内经四季养生法 [M]. 北京：中国中医药出版社，2009.

Xu Wenbing. *Health Nurturing in Four Seasons of Huangdi Neijing*[M]. Beijing: China Press of Traditional Chinese Medicine, 2009.

烟建华.《难经》理论与实践 [M]. 北京：人民卫生出版社，2005.

Yan Jianhua. *Theories and Practices of Nanjing*[M]. Beijing: People's Medical Publishing House, 2005.

正安棠. 2018 养生手账 [M]. 北京：人民卫生出版社，2017.

Zheng Antang. *2018 Records of Health Nurturing*[M]. Beijing: People's Medical Publishing House, 2017.

张树生. 神农本草经理论与实践 [M]. 北京：人民卫生出版社，2010.

Zhang Shusheng. *Theories and Practices of Shennong Bencao Jing*[M]. Beijing: People's Medical Publishing House, 2010.

附录 1: 二十四节气
Annex 1: Twenty-four Solar Terms

24 Solar Terms	二十四节气	二十四节气（拼音）24 Solar Terms (Pinyin)	日期 Dates	太阳黄经 Sun's Ecliptic Longitude
Beginning of Spring	立春	lì chūn	Feb 5th	315°
Rain Water	雨水	yǔ shuǐ	Feb 19th	330°
Insects Awakening	惊蛰	jīng zhé	March 6th	345°
Spring Equinox	春分	chūn fēn	March 21st	0°
Fresh Green	清明	qīng míng	April 5th	15°
Grain Rain	谷雨	gǔ yǔ	April 20th	30°
Beginning of Summer	立夏	lì xià	May 6th	45°
Lesser Fullness	小满	xiǎo mǎn	May 21st	60°
Grain in Ear	芒种	máng zhòng	June 6th	75°
Summer Solstice	夏至	xià zhì	June 21st	90°
Lesser Heat	小暑	xiǎo shǔ	July 7th	105°
Greater Heat	大暑	dà shǔ	July 23th	120°
Beginning of Autumn	立秋	lì qiū	Aug 8th	135°
End of Heat	处暑	chù shǔ	Aug 23rd	150°
White Dew	白露	bái lù	Sep 8th	165°
Autumn Equinox	秋分	qiū fēn	Sep 23rd	180°
Cold Dew	寒露	hán lù	Oct 9th	195°
First Frost	霜降	shuāng jiàng	Oct 24th	210°
Beginning of Winter	立冬	lì dōng	Nov 8th	225°
Light Snow	小雪	xiǎo xuě	Nov 23rd	240°
Heavy Snow	大雪	dà xuě	Dec 7th	255°
Winter Solstice	冬至	dōng zhì	Dec 22nd	270°
Lesser Cold	小寒	xiǎo hán	Jan 6th	285°
Greater Cold	大寒	dà hán	Jan 20th	300°

附录 2：二十四节气养生食疗方
Annex 2: Health-nurturing Recipes in 24 Solar Terms

Recipe	食疗方	对应节气 Corresponding Solar Term	页码 Page
Stewed Carrots and Beef	胡萝卜炖牛肉	立春(Beginning of Spring)	18
Pueraria Root and Prepared Soybean Porridge	粉葛豆豉粥	雨水(Rain Water)	22
Spring Bamboo Shoots and Ribbonfish Soup	带鱼春笋汤	惊蛰(Insects Awakening)	26
Yam and Walnut Paste	山药核桃羹	春分(Spring Equinox)	30
Crispy Fried Yam	香酥山药	清明(Fresh Green)	34
Rib Soup with White Gourd, Kelp, and Lotus Leaves	冬瓜海带荷叶排骨汤	谷雨(Grain Rain)	37
Sponge Gourd Porridge	丝瓜粥	立夏(Beginning of Summer)	54
Soy Milk of Pearl Barley, Mung Bean and Red Bean	薏仁红绿豆浆	小满(Lesser Fullness)	57
Steamed Egg Custard with Fresh Lotus Root Juice	鲜藕蛋羹	芒种(Grain in Ear)	61

Recipe	食疗方	对应节气 Corresponding Solar Term	页码 Page
Porridge of Pearl Barley and Mung Bean	薏仁绿豆粥	夏至(Summer Solstice)	63
Stewed Pork with Lotus Seeds and Lily	莲子百合煨猪肉	小暑(Lesser Heat)	69
Porridge of Lotus Leaves and Mint	荷叶薄荷粥	大暑(Greater Heat)	74
Lily Almond Porridge	百合杏仁粥	立秋(Beginning of Autumn)	91
Adenophora Porridge	沙参粥	处暑(End of Heat)	108
Stewed Chicken with Astragalus and Notoginseng	黄芪三七鸡	白露(White Dew)	98
Asparagus Porridge	天门冬粥	秋分(Autumn Equinox)	102
Stewed Snow Pear with Sichuan Scallop	川贝炖雪梨	寒露(Cold Dew)	105
Chestnut Porridge	栗子粥	霜降(First Frost)	108
Ten Powerful Tonics Decoction	十全大补汤	立冬(Beginning of Winter)	123
Stewed Beef with Astragalus and Longan	黄芪桂圆牛肉汤	小雪(Light Snow)	127

Recipe	食疗方	对应节气 Corresponding Solar Term	页码 Page
Mixed Mashed Garlic and Crown Daisy	蒜泥茼蒿	大雪(Heavy Snow)	130
Stewed Mutton with Daikon	白萝卜炖羊肉	冬至(Winter Solstice)	134
Stewed Mutton with Chinese angelica and Ginger	当归生姜羊肉汤	小寒(Lesser Cold)	137
Stewed Poussin with Astragalus and Chinese Wolfberry	黄芪枸杞炖童子鸡	大寒(Greater Cold)	143
Snow Fungus and Chinese Wolfberry Soup	银耳枸杞汤	提高免疫力食疗方(Health—nurtur—ing Recipe for Enhancing Immunity)	148
Astragalus and Jujube Tea	黄芪红枣茶	提高免疫力食疗方(Health—nurtur—ing Recipe for Enhancing Immunity)	149
American ginseng and Lean meat Porridge	西洋参瘦肉粥	提高免疫力食疗方(Health—nurtur—ing Recipe for Enhancing Immunity)	150

附录 3：食物和药材
Annex 3: Food and Medicinals

食物或药材	Food or Medicinals
（淡）豆豉	prepared soybean (Dan Douchi)
八角	star anise
白菜	Chinese cabbage
白参	white ginseng (Baishen)
白酒	Chinese baijiu
白萝卜	daikon
白（砂）糖	white sugar
白芍	debark peony root (Baishao)
白术	largehead atractylodes rhizome (Baizhu)
蚌肉	mussels
薄荷	mint
扁豆	lentil
冰糖	rock sugar
菠菜	spinach
鲳鱼	butterfish
赤小豆	red beans
川贝	Sichuan scallop (Chuanbei)
川芎	Sichuan lovage rhizome (Chuanxiong)
葱	green onion
大葱	leek
大麦	barley
当归	Chinese angelica (Danggui)

食物或药材	Food or Medicinals
党参	tangshen (Dangshen)
淀粉	starch
冬虫夏草	Chinese caterpillar fungus (Dongchongxiacao)
冬瓜	white gourd
食物或药材	Food or Medicinals
冬笋	winter bamboo shoots
冬小麦	winter wheat
豆腐	tofu
肥母鸡	poulard
粉葛	pueraria root
茯苓	indian bread (Fuling)
甘草	liquorice
甘蔗	sugarcane
柑橘	citrus fruits
枸杞（子）	Chinese wolfberry
桂花	osmanthus blossoms
桂皮	cinnamon
桂圆	Longan
桂枝	cassia twig (Guizhi)
海带	kelp
荷叶	lotus leaves
核桃	walnut
黑豆	black soybean
红参	red ginseng (Hongshen)

食物或药材	Food or Medicinals
红椒	red pepper
红薯	sweet potato
红糖	brown sugar
红枣	jujube
胡椒粉	pepper
花椒	Sichuan pepper
花生	peanut
山（药）	Henan yam
黄（花）鱼	yellow croaker
食物或药材	Food or Medicinals
黄酒	yellow rice wine (Huangjiu)
黄芪	astragalus (Huangqi)
茴香	fennel
鸡精	chicken powder
荠菜	shepherd's purse
鲫鱼	crucian carp
姜	ginger
酱油	soy sauce
芥菜	leaf mustard
芥末	mustard
金银花露	Honeysuckle Tea
金针菇	enokitake
粳米	japonica rice (Jingmi)
韭菜	Chinese chives

食物或药材	Food or Medicinals
菊花茶	Chrysanthemum Tea
苦瓜	bitter gourd
栗子	chestnut
莲藕	lotus root
莲子	lotus seeds
莲子心	lotus plumule
芦根	reed rhizome (Lugen)
萝卜	radish
萝卜子	radish seed
绿豆	mung bean
绿豆汤	Mung Bean Soup
麦冬	ophiopogon tuber (Maidong)
米醋	rice vinegar
墨鱼	cuttlefish
食物或药材	Food or Medicinals
木耳	wood ear
木通	akebia stem (Mutong)
排骨	pork ribs
芹菜	celery
人参	ginseng
人丹	Rendan Pills
肉桂	cassia bark (Rougui)
三七	notoginseng (Sanqi)
沙参	adenophora root (Shashen)

食物或药材	Food or Medicinals
山药	yam
山楂	Chinese hawthorn fruit
山竹	mangosteen
芍药	Chinese peony (Shaoyao)
石榴	pomegranate
柿子	persimmon
首乌	fleeceflower root (Shouwu)
熟地	prepared rehmannia root (Shudi)
丝瓜	sponge gourd
酸梅汤	Sour Plum Drink
蒜	garlic
蒜泥	mashed garlic
桃子	peach
天（门）冬	asparagus (Tian<men>dong)
茼蒿	crown daisy
童子鸡	poussin
娃娃菜	baby cabbage
豌豆苗	pea sprout
味精	MSG (monosodium glutamate)
食物或药材	Food or Medicinals
莴苣	stem lettuce
乌梅	smoked plum
五味子	chinese magnoliavine fruit (Wuweizi)
细辛	manchurian wildginger root (Xixin)

食物或药材	Food or Medicinals
西洋参	American ginseng
咸肉	salt meat
香椿	Chinese toon sprouts (Xiangchun)
香菇	shiitake
香瓜	muskmelon
香油	sesame oil
小米	millet
杏	apricot
杏仁	almonds
雪梨	snow bear
薏仁	pearl barley
银耳（白木耳）	snow fungus
柚子	pomelo
柚子	pomelo
芋头	taro
芝麻	sesame
植物油	vegetable oil
肘子	ham hock
猪肚	pork tripe
猪肝	pork liver
竹笋	bamboo shoot

附录 4：穴位名
Annex 4: Acupoints

穴位名	Acupoints	页码 Page
涌泉	Yongquan (KI 1)	7
大敦	Dadun (LR 1)	13
太冲	Taichong (LR 3)	14
肝俞	Ganshu (BL 18)	15
膻中	Danzhong (CV 17)	50
至阳	Zhiyang (GV 9)	51
内关	Neiguan (PC 6)	52
足三里	Zusanli (ST 36)	57
迎香	Yingxiang (LI 20)	85
肺俞	Feishu (BL 13)	86
列缺	Lieque (LU 7)	87
气海	Qihai (CV 6)	119
太溪	Taixi (KI 3)	120